# Therapeutic Exercise for Spinal Segmental Stabilization in Low Back Pain

For Churchill Livingstone

*Editorial Director:* Mary Law
*Design Direction:* Judith Wright

# Therapeutic Exercise for Spinal Segmental Stabilization in Low Back Pain

## Scientific Basis and Clinical Approach

**Carolyn Richardson** PhD BPhty (Hons)
Associate Professor and Reader, Department of Physiotherapy, University of Queensland, Australia

**Gwendolen Jull** MPhty, GradDipManipTher FACP
Associate Professor and Reader, Department of Physiotherapy, University of Queensland, Australia

**Paul Hodges** PhD BPhty (Hons)
NHMRC Postdoctoral Research Fellow, Prince of Wales Medical Research Institute, Sydney, Australia

**Julie Hides** PhD MPhtyST BPhty
Clinical Supervisor, Joint Stability Assessment Clinic, Department of Physiotherapy, University of Queensland, Australia


Foreword by

**Manohar M Panjabi** PhD DTech
Professor, Department of Orthopaedics and Rehabilitation, Yale University School of Medicine, New Haven, CT USA

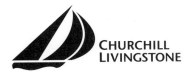

CHURCHILL
LIVINGSTONE

EDINBURGH LONDON NEW YORK PHILADELPHIA SYDNEY AND TORONTO 1999

First published 1999

ISBN 0 443 058024

**British Library Cataloguing in Publication Data**
A catalogue record for this book is available from the British
Library.

**Library of Congress Cataloging in Publication Data**
A catalog record for this book is available from the Library of
Congress.

**Note**
Medical knowledge is constantly changing. As new
information becomes available, changes in treatment,
procedures, equipment and the use of drugs become
necessary. The authors and the publishers have, as far as it
is possible, taken care to ensure that the information given in
this text is accurate and up to date. However, readers are
strongly advised to confirm that the information, especially
with regard to drug usage, complies with latest legislation
and standards of practice.

The
publisher's
policy is to use
**paper manufactured
from sustainable forests**

Printed in the United Kingdom

# Contents

# Foreword

You all have heard the story of four blind men who were asked to examine an elephant. The one touching the legs said that it was the trunk of a tree. The other, who held the elephant's trunk in his hands, was certain that it was a rubber hose. The third one felt the sharp bristles of the tail and pronounced it to be a bottlebrush. The fourth, who was touching the large ears, thought them to be fans. Thus all four descriptions were truthful but none identified the animal.

Clinical spinal instability is like an elephant. Even though we know its manifestations, still we do not fully understand it. An engineer thinks of it as a mechanical structure that has become mechanically unstable. An orthopaedic surgeon has a different viewpoint. She or he thinks of it as a mechanical structure that has lost its ability to maintain the normal physiological patterns of motion, resulting in clinical symptoms of pain and/or neurological dysfunction. A physical therapist may diagnose the problem as the deficiency in the muscular part of the spinal stabilizing system. While a more severe condition may require complete elimination of motion at the sight of injury or dysfunction by fusion surgery, the lesser instability may be suitably treated with muscle alterations leading to decreased spinal motion. The human spine is a remarkable structure, performing seemingly conflicting functions: carrying large spinal loads, allowing motions in multiple planes between body parts, and protecting the delicate spinal cord and nerve roots. Mechanical stability, both static and dynamic, is needed to perform these fundamental functions. As the osteoligamentous spine can carry only a fraction of the actual loads to which the spine is subjected in daily living, the importance of the spinal muscles and their control becomes obvious.

The authors of this book have produced a text that focuses on the spinal muscles, specifically on their potential to stabilize the spinal column. There is significant biomechanical literature describing the role of various anatomical components on the stability of the spinal column, but this is not the case for the muscles. The studies about the role of muscles on spinal stability are few. There are inherent difficulties in studying the biomechanical role of muscles *in vivo*. The authors have made significant research contributions in this field. In this text, they not only present their own and others' research on the potential for the spinal muscles and their neural control to stabilize the spine, but also clearly present the hypothesis of the spinal stabilizing system, and, most importantly, their clinical experience in helping the low back pain patient by using their methodology.

This text, to my knowledge, is a first of its kind that attempts to synthesize the available information about the dynamic stabilization of the spinal column by spinal musculature, especially as it relates to the low back pain problem. The book is a well-conceived bridge between the basic research and clinical practice. It should be of significant interest to physical and occupational therapists and other professionals who clinically deal with the problems of the low back. It may even help better identify the animal of clinical instability.

1998                                                    M.M.P

# Preface

Therapeutic exercise to restore muscle function is an integrated part of the body of knowledge which constitutes physical therapy. In the past it may have been said that therapeutic exercise to restore muscle function in back pain sufferers was more of an art, where treatment was given on a trial and error basis with no clear understanding of why some exercises seemed more effective than others. The approach to therapeutic exercise for low back pain described in this book evolved from an early idea, gained from research and treatment in physical therapy, that some muscles have a primary function for support and protection of joints. This idea was expanded into a new way of thinking about exercise to prevent low back pain recurring or indeed occurring in the first place.

While research is the cornerstone for a greater understanding of therapeutic exercise, initially the primary challenge was devising the relevant research questions that would unlock the mysteries of the problems in the muscles of back pain patients. The key to the new discoveries has been the close link between clinicians and researchers in an upward spiral of discovery with one step ventured by innovative clinical work, the next by innovative scientific discoveries. As each cycle repeated itself, the knowledge base gradually grew. This process has developed from the mutual recognition by clinicians and researchers of each other's particular talents.

This spiral of discovery has brought together the work of many astute clinicians and innovative scientists. The result is the development of a new type of exercise for the management of low back pain sufferers, which is presented in this book. *Spinal segmental stabilization* is an innovative method of delivering therapeutic exercise to the patient. In many ways it is the antithesis to traditional exercise methods such as strength and endurance training, which have formed the basis for the therapeutic exercise for musculoskeletal conditions for so long. *Spinal segmental stabilization* is designed to specifically improve the underlying joint stabilization rather than training functional movement and hoping joint control improves concurrently.

Changing traditional thinking about the exercise treatment of a common problem such as back pain is always difficult. The enormous challenge to effect change was the stimulus that led to the writing of this text and allowed us to present our ideas for evaluation. Only time will tell if a change in thinking does occur and if this book does fulfil its role in developing physical therapy treatments and in fostering and stimulating further research.

The discovery of motor control problems in back pain patients and the subsequent developments of new measures of these muscle problems have given the opportunity to effect change in another way. In an era where accountability is important, physical therapists must embrace the concept that it is not enough that patients believe they are improving with treatment. The way in which they have benefited from physical therapy should be measurable by objective tests that assess the way physical treatment is changing their physical condition. Tests that reflect change as a result of therapeutic exercise to enhance joint stabilization have not been available. This book includes the first of these measures, with the hope that further research and clinical endeavours will see them evolve as standard procedures acknowledged by the physical therapy and medical professions as being appropriate and relevant for evaluating their patients' progress.

Technology is playing an increasingly important role in both the treatment and assessment of the deep muscles. While it is essential that the physical therapy profession improve their understanding of the skeletal muscle system and embraces highly technical equipment such as real time ultrasound imaging, it is also vital that these skills are introduced appropriately. Modalities such as real time ultrasound should not be seen as a substitute for high levels of clinical skill but rather should be introduced as an adjunct to physical treatment modalities.

What is the future? Now that the function of the deep muscles have been discovered and specific exercises devised to target them in rehabilitation, one vital question remains. In some circumstances, can less specific exercises also change the motor control problems in back pain patients? While we do not believe this is so, it remains an important research question for physical therapists as well as for many other health care professionals and is the focus of our continuing research efforts.

As four good friends we have enjoyed this voyage of discovery and look forward to working together for many years to come in developing and furthering our knowledge of *Spinal segmental stabilization*.

1998

C.R.
G.J.
P.H.
J.H.

# Acknowledgements

There are many people we need to thank. From the Department of Physiotherapy, The University of Queensland, Quentin Scott, Sue Roll and all in the Back Pain Assessment Clinic for their constant enthusiasm. They have made a significant contribution to the development of the new clinical skills, which are described in this book. Joseph Ng and Christine Hamilton contributed to the developing knowledge in the early years and helped us develop a broader perspective on the muscle dysfunction and exercise treatments associated with low back pain. We are grateful for their help and friendship. Associate Professor Yvonne Burns, Head of the Department showed faith in our research and was a source of continued encouragement. We would particularly like to acknowledge her help in the formation and development of the Clinic, and also Dr Tony Wright for his help in acquiring real time ultrasound imaging for the assessments.

Our knowledge of real time ultrasound imaging was only possible through the assistance, instruction and encouragement of Dr David Cooper, an obstetrician who specializes in the use of real time ultrasound imaging. He is assisting in guiding its introduction into physical therapy practice. We thank Dr Vaughan Kippers of the Anatomy Department, The University of Queensland for help in our studies of the deep muscles and for assistance with many of the cadaveric dissections illustrated in this book. In addition, the collaboration of Professor Simon Gandevia, from the Prince of Wales Medical Research Institute, and Professor Alf Thorstensson and Dr Andrew Cresswell from the Karolinska Institute, Sweden in the development of many of the scientific questions was greatly appreciated.

We also thank Wendy Sparkes who enthusiastically took on the role of helping us prepare the manuscript. We really appreciated her attention to detail which allowed us to finally finish the book. Finally and most importantly we could not have developed and then written about our ideas for exercise if it had not been for the encouragement, patience and understanding of our friends and family. Thanks to everyone.

# Introduction

SECTION CONTENTS

# The reason for change

It is well known that the lifetime incidence of low back pain is extraordinarily high, but those who incur the majority of the cost, both personally and financially, are the persons who suffer recurrent and persistent or chronic pain. Manipulative or manual therapy is one of the fundamental treatment methods used by physical therapists, osteopaths, chiropractors and manual medicine practitioners in the management of low back pain. There is evidence that manipulative therapy can be effective for the relief of pain and restoration of motion in the short term,[14,192,304] but this therapy has not met the challenge of lessening persistent and recurrent episodes of low back pain. This was also our clinical experience and, in addition, general back exercises appeared to have equal limitations for the goal of controlling pain and preventing recurrent or persistent episodes of pain.[194]

Stabilization programmes attracted our interest, with their aims of using the muscle system to protect spinal joint structures from further repetitive microtrauma, recurrent pain and degenerative change.[181,288,292,293] Our research experience with the knee musculature suggested to us that the exercises in many of the stabilization programmes were not specific enough. Studies of the normal knee indicated that some muscles were controlling and supporting joint position, while other muscles were more concerned with producing joint movement.[279] In the pathological knee, it was found that the muscles controlling and supporting the position of the joint were those which were predominantly dysfunctional. While addressing issues such as neutral joint postures and muscle co-contraction for joint support, low back stabilization programmes did not focus on those muscles most likely to protect individual spinal joints and did not consider that deficits may be present in particular muscles and not in others.

This book describes specific stabilizing exercises that are based on the impairment found in particular muscles of back pain patients, and a method of exercise which will ensure their functional return. This new direction in therapeutic exercise for spinal joint stabilization has been developed over several years, its development involving clinical problem solving and technical skills as well as basic and applied scientific research. It was initially through studying how the muscles could provide lumbar segmental stabilization that insight was gained into the type of therapeutic exercise that may be beneficial for supporting the spinal joints, controlling pain and preventing recurrent bouts of low back pain.

The biomechanical research by Panjabi[262–264] and others introduced a new framework for a more comprehensive interpretation and understanding of spinal stabilization, clinical instability and its relationship to back pain. Rather than limiting the definition of instability to an osseoligamentous insufficiency resulting in abnormally large and pathological intersegmental displacements, spinal stabilization is viewed as the composite function of three systems, the osseoligamentous system, the muscle system and the neural control system. This model highlights the important role of muscles, especially the small intrinsic muscles of the spine, as well as their neural control for segmental stabilization. Breakdown in either the muscles themselves or in the manner in which their activity is controlled and regulated, as well as inadequacies in the passive osseoligamentous structures, can constitute a spinal stabilization problem, which can cause or perpetuate low back pain.

The link between spinal stabilization and low back pain raised important issues in relation to stabilization exercises:

- What muscles were most important for spinal segmental support?

- Were these muscles operating in their supporting role in back pain patients?
- Could dysfunctional muscles be retrained to regain their supporting role?
- Could muscles be trained to compensate for impaired passive support?

In overviewing the stabilizing role of the trunk and back muscles our attention became focused on muscles which controlled the lumbar and lumbosacral joints rather than on muscles which span the spine from the thorax to pelvis. It was considered that muscles such as the lumbar multifidus, transversus abdominis, and possibly also parts of the obliquus internus abdominis, would most likely function to stabilize the segments of the lumbar spine. In order to check if these muscles were functioning in low back pain patients, it was necessary to devise specific muscle tests.

Drawing in of the abdominal wall is a manoeuvre that has been described by Kendall & McCreary[180] as one that activates the oblique abdominal muscles. While some contraction of the oblique muscles would be expected, Strohl et al,[325] Lacôte et al[202] and, later, DeTroyer et al[83] described the action of 'pulling the belly in' as one in which the transversus abdominis predominated. We adopted the motor skill of drawing in the abdominal wall as the test of the function of the deep abdominal muscles. Performance of tasks such as a sit-up provides indications of the strength and endurance of the entire abdominal muscle group but does not indicate the specific function of the transversus abdominis. An air-filled pressure device (pressure biofeedback unit) was developed to meet the challenge of gaining some quantification of this deep muscle action.[176,281,283] A clinical test to assess the action of the segmental lumbar multifidus became another challenge. Lumbar extension tests the entire erector spinae muscle group (including thoracic portions), but does not give an indication of the local function of its segmentally arranged fascicles.[230] An isometric test was devised which involved the action of slowly activating the muscle under the guidance of the therapist's fingers. The feature of this test

was that a co-contraction of the deep abdominals was observed. It was reasoned that the
observation of this deep muscle interaction had
potentially considerable functional significance,
as the co-contraction of these muscles on each
side of the spine would be able to increase the
stiffness of the lumbar segments without inter-
fering with trunk movement.

The development of specific tests to target the
stabilization function of particular muscles for
the clinical situation was a considerable step
forward. It introduced, for the first time, tests
that addressed a previously uninvestigated
muscle function, and which could be added to
the current musculoskeletal assessment of low
back pain patients. Clinical use of these tests of
transversus abdominis and lumbar multifidus
muscle function quickly indicated that patients
with back pain had difficulties in performance
that are not so evident in persons who have
never suffered from back pain. In an early pilot
trial, a clinician with experience of the clinical
test of transversus abdominis used the pressure
biofeedback unit to assess a group of non-back-
pain subjects and a group of back pain patients
in a single-blind manner.[282] This pilot study lent
support to clinical observations, and revealed
that only 10% of those with a history of low back
pain could perform the transversus abdominis
test, compared with 82% of the non-low-back-
pain subjects. Interestingly, the test result
appeared to be independent of age or gender.
This pilot study gave some preliminary evidence
that the presence of transversus abdominis
dysfunction might discriminate between those
persons with and those without a history of low
back pain.

The exercise skills involved in these clinical
tests became the basis of our specific exercise
programmes for improving spinal segmental
stiffness. Clinically, improvement in the ability
to perform and hold the deep muscle co-
contraction was found to be closely linked to
patients' reports of reduction in pain levels,
expressions that the back felt safer and the
ability of patients to control their back pain. The
development of an exercise programme that
seemed to assist most back pain patients led to

the formation of two research streams. One
involved clinical trials to investigate the efficacy
of the specific exercise approach. The other
involved mechanism studies addressing the
issues of how these particular deep muscles
stabilized the spine, as well as determining the
precise nature of the muscle dysfunction in back
pain patients.

Two prospective, randomized, controlled
clinical trials were conducted independently of
our group on chronic low back pain patients to
investigate the efficacy of this specific exercise
programme.[257,259] Patient groups in each trial
had a diagnosed pathology of clinical instability,
the first study group with radiological evidence
of spondylolysis and spondylolisthesis and the
second without any bony defect. These trials
demonstrated that the 10-week specific exercise
programme significantly decreased pain and
increased functional ability in the treatment
groups. There was virtually no change in pain or
function in the control groups, who received
conventional conservative treatments, including
exercise such as swimming, gym work and sit-
ups. With respect to the long-term effect of the
specific exercise, the trial group of patients with
spondylolysis and spondylolisthesis were shown
to have maintained their improvement at the 30-
month follow-up. Follow-up of the second
patient group is in progress. It could be argued
that the sustained pain relief and the increased
functional levels achieved by the specific
exercise group could indicate that the particular
muscles capable of controlling the lumbar
segment had been trained to compensate for the
impaired passive joint structures.

Further information on the mechanisms of
how the specific exercise training affects back
pain, disability and recurrence rate has been
gained from another randomized, controlled,
clinical trial which examined first-episode acute
unilateral low back pain patients.[136] These back
pain patients had no demonstrable bony
pathology on a plain radiograph but, irrespective
of the nature of the onset of their back pain, all
demonstrated a reduction in the cross-sectional
area of the lumbar multifidus at the segment
and side of pain on ultrasound imaging. This

reduction in size is consistent with pain and reflex inhibition of the segmental muscle. The treatment group undertook the specific exercise training involving co-contraction of transversus abdominis and lumbar multifidus over a 4-week period. These patients demonstrated an increase in cross-sectional area of the affected multifidus, its cross-sectional area returning to equal that of the non-symptomatic side. The control group who did not receive the specific exercise but who had medical management only and were encouraged to resume normal activity, did not demonstrate any improvement in the cross-sectional areas of their impaired segmental multifidus muscle over the 4-week period. Most importantly, it was shown that the exercise group who were able to restore their lumbar multifidus size had a significantly lower recurrence rate of low back pain episodes compared with the control group in the year following initial injury.[133,137] This study demonstrated that the specific exercise technique could change an impaired muscle. With the positive long-term outcome of the treatment group, it seems that the multifidus muscle (and probably transversus abdominis, although not measured) had been retrained to contribute again to joint support.

While the main focus of these clinical trials was to demonstrate the efficacy of the specific exercise treatment compared with other types of conservative management, they contributed to knowledge of how the exercise could have resulted in beneficial effects in the back pain patients. Nevertheless, more detailed studies were required, especially of the transversus abdominis and the oblique abdominal muscles, in order to determine the exact nature of the problem in these muscles in low back pain patients. Equally, it was necessary to study how an exercise which is so specific (i.e. exercising some muscles without their synergists working) could affect and alleviate the muscle impairments.

The answers to these questions are emerging largely from the research being done by Hodges and others. A fundamental discovery was that the muscle dysfunction in low back pain was a problem in motor control in the deep muscles related to segmental joint stabilization. Normally, in its spinal supporting role, the transversus abdominis appears to be controlled independently of the other abdominal muscles. Its action is closely linked to that of the diaphragm and pelvic floor muscles, and appears to affect spinal support through its attachments to the thoracolumbar fascia and its close links to the development of intra-abdominal pressure. Its contraction with the deep fibres of lumbar multifidus during normal function, of which we have preliminary clinical and laboratory evidence, has allowed us to put forward a case for these muscles forming a deep abdominal corset controlling the lumbo pelvic joints during dynamic and static functional tasks. This pattern of motor control is lost in low back pain patients. Future studies on transversus abdominis using various experimental paradigms will undoubtedly shed more light on these motor control problems.

The studies completed to date within these two areas of research have given us confidence to suggest that these specific exercises are essential in the treatment of low back pain to gain long-term pain relief for this common musculoskeletal complaint. The research has allowed us to refine and modify our original exercise strategies in line with the findings of motor control deficits in key muscles for stabilization. The exercise strategies described aim to give clinicians methods to help patients relearn a motor skill required for joint support with the objective of re-establishing effective automatic motor patterns.

This book presents the basic and clinical science on which the exercises for the motor control deficits were developed, and describes in detail a new evidence-based treatment approach to the problem of low back pain. Knowledge of the mechanisms of function and dysfunction has also guided the development of assessment techniques for the motor control deficits in the deep muscles. These emerging methods of invasive laboratory tests, as well as non-invasive clinical assessments of motor control problems, are presented. These are likely to rapidly advance our knowledge of the neural control mechanisms involved in the stabilization of the spine. In addition, the development of non-invasive clinical tests has led to the recognition of the often individual nature of each patient's motor control problems. This has guided more efficient and optimal methods of retraining the motor patterns required for joint support. These non-invasive measures have laid the foundation for a problem-solving process in therapeutic exercise for spinal segmental stabilization. Therapeutic exercise thus not only becomes a clinical skill but also moves towards becoming a more exacting clinical science.

# The scientific basis

Controlled scientific experimentation is required to identify how the muscular control system is affected in the low back pain patient and how specific exercise treatments can affect change in these impairments. This section provides discussion of the current state of evidence at this point. The focus of this discussion is the deep segmental stabilizing system of the spine.

# 2

# Back pain and lumbopelvic stabilization: the case for the local muscle system

Stabilization of the lumbar spine is a complex issue. The study of biomechanical and neurophysiological models in relation to spinal stability has developed as a major research focus in the continuing search towards understanding the factors that contribute to, and the treatment of, low back pain. This chapter explores a link between back pain and lumbopelvic stabilization and considers the role of the muscles concerned with spinal stabilization. Through such attention, some of the directions of therapeutic exercise for the treatment of the low back pain patient are established.

The maintenance of spinal stability encompasses three main elements: the passive support of the osseoligamentous structures, the support of the muscle system, and control of the muscle system by the central nervous system. Two interrelated parameters of spinal stability need to be considered due to the multisegmental nature of the lumbar spine. The first parameter is control of spinal orientation, which relates to the maintenance of the overall posture of the spine against imposed forces and compressive loading. The second is control of the intersegmental relationship at the local level (i.e. lumbar segmental control), irrespective of changes in the overall orientation of the spine. Efficient stability of the spine is dependent on the integrity of both levels of support.[106] The two parameters are interdependent and yet have independent characteristics for their united purpose of the control and protection of the lumbar spine and neural elements during daily function. Strategies for control of spinal orientation are linked to the direction and distribution of the external forces acting on the spine.[33] Control of the lumbar segment and maintenance of a stable relationship between adjacent vertebrae is more complex. Each lumbar motion segment has six degrees of freedom, with rotations and translations occurring around three mutually perpendicular axes,[351] presenting a system with potentially a large amount of redundancy that requires control to allow effective function.[183] It would seem that it is the challenge to control the intersegmental relationship or, in other words, to maintain sufficient intervertebral stiffness[33] for normal pain-free function, which is one of the key issues in the production and perpetuation, and thus the management, of mechanical low back pain.

## SPINAL STABILIZATION

In the clinical sense spinal stability and, conversely, spinal instability are terms and conditions that have led to considerable debate among the medical and bioengineering fraternities.[18,33,36,102,106,108,272] Difficulties lie, particularly in vivo, in gaining a definition of instability that would indicate a relationship to a pain state and that would generate a method of quantification to demonstrate its presence. As a consequence, there is currently neither a gold-standard definition of clinical instability nor a gold-standard measure.[37]

Panjabi[262] introduced an innovative model of the spinal stabilization system which serves as an appropriate model for understanding the entity of spinal stability and instability and fits the clinical paradigm for the assessment and treatment of the muscle dysfunction in the low back pain patient. The model incorporates a passive subsystem, an active subsystem and a neural control subsystem (Fig. 2.1). The passive subsystem incorporates the osseous and articular structures and the spinal ligaments, and their control of segmental movement, not only at end of range, but particularly around the neutral joint position. While being integral components of the spinal stabilization system, the spinal ligaments offer most restraint towards the end

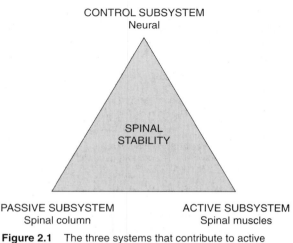

CONTROL SUBSYSTEM
Neural

SPINAL
STABILITY

PASSIVE SUBSYSTEM          ACTIVE SUBSYSTEM
Spinal column              Spinal muscles

**Figure 2.1**   The three systems that contribute to active spinal stabilization. (Adapted from Panjabi[262].)

of the range of movement, but do not provide substantial support in neutral joint postures. The active subsystem refers to the force-generating capacity of the muscles themselves, which provides the mechanical ability to stabilize the spinal segment. The control of these muscles for the requirement of spinal support is described as the neural control subsystem. This model recognizes that muscles need to be programmed, in response to feedback (e.g. from sensory cues from ligaments), in order to adjust to any condition at any point in time so that the appropriate muscles are activated to the appropriate level. Based on this model, Panjabi[262] contends that the three subsystems are interdependent components of the spinal stabilization system with one capable of compensating for deficits in another. Back pain can occur as a consequence of deficits in control of the spinal segment when abnormally large segmental motions cause compression or stretch on neural structures or abnormal deformation of ligaments and pain-sensitive structures.[263] These deficits may potentially be caused by a dysfunction in any of the three systems, which cannot be compensated for by the other systems.

What constitutes instability at the segmental level has been a point of debate, and it has been variously defined as a loss of joint stiffness,[106,272] an increase in mobility and abnormal spinal motion,[103] and changes in the ratios of segmental rotations and translations.[350] Traditionally, instability has been more aligned with the presence of abnormal motion at the end-point of the range, even though instability has long been associated with degenerative disease where the segment may exhibit lesser total motion. In contrast, Panjabi's[262] hypothesis identifies control of intersegmental motion around the neutral zone as a major parameter of spinal instability involved in the mechanism of clinical instability. The load–deformation behaviour of the spinal segment is non-linear and is highly flexible in the vicinity of the neutral position. This is the region known as the neutral zone[262] (Fig. 2.2). Motion occurs in this region of the physiological intervertebral motion against minimal internal resistance, with the ligamentous structures providing restraint in the elastic zone to limit end range of motion. The neutral zone presents a specific problem to the spinal stability mechanism, and there is evidence supporting its contribution to clinical instability. Injuring the spine in vitro by dividing ligaments or the disc or removing the posterior spinal elements results in potentially multidirectional instabilities and an increase in both the neutral zone and physiological range of motion.[3,265] In a study subjecting porcine cervical spines to high-speed trauma, the neutral zone was found to increase to a greater extent than the range of motion, and also to be the first indicator of the onset of injury.[260] In a pivotal study which suggests a link between excessive neutral zone motion and pain, the effect of external fixation of the cervical segment was evaluated. This technique is used clinically to evaluate the effect of fixation on the likely control of spinal pain as a prognostic indicator for treatment by spinal fusion. When the technique was applied to cadaveric cervical spine specimens, the motion parameter that decreased the most was the neutral zone (71%, compared to a 38% decrease in the total range of motion).[262] This evidence of the sensitivity of and increase in the neutral zone relating to spinal instability has led to a new definition of clinical instability:

*Clinical instability: A significant decrease in the capacity of the stabilizing system of the spine to maintain the intervertebral neutral zones within physiological limits which results in pain and disability.* (Panjabi,[262] p. 394).

While the concept of the neutral zone was developed from studying passive structures, it is the contribution of active muscle contraction or muscle tone in relation to the control of the neutral zone that links this theory to the real-life situation. The ligaments and other passive structures can only provide support towards the end of the range. Instability within this broader definition, which encompasses three interrelated systems, may therefore relate also to insufficiency of the muscle system.[263] Decreased muscle stiffness resulting from fatigue, degenerative changes or injury may lead to spinal instability.[106] Furthermore, damage to spinal structures may result from insufficient muscle control to maintain stability at either or both levels of spinal postural control and or control at the intersegmental level.[106] Conversely, the muscle system also has the potential to compensate for instability by increasing the stiffness of the lumbar spine and decreasing the size of the neutral zone.[54,106,263]

This link between muscle function and spinal stiffness and the neutral zone provides the basis of the possible conservative management, through therapeutic exercise, of spinal instability. To investigate this link further, a more detailed

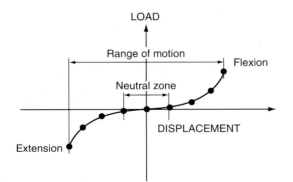

**Figure 2.2** Schematic representation of the load–deformation behaviour of the spinal segment highlighting the region known as the neutral zone. (Reproduced with permission from Panjabi.[264])

understanding of the muscle system (i.e. the active subsystem and the neural control system) is required.

## MUSCLE FUNCTION IN SPINAL SEGMENTAL STABILIZATION

Muscular stabilization of the spine has always been recognized as important in human function. All skeletal muscles of the trunk and pelvic region contribute to some extent to stabilization of the spinal joints. Arguments are presented here to explain why our focus for rehabilitation of low back pain has been on some particular muscles of the spine and not others.

### The concept of muscles designed for spinal segmental support

The first suggestion that some muscles surrounding the spine are primarily concerned with stability is ascribed to Leonardo Da Vinci.[68] In describing muscles of the neck, he suggested that the more central muscles stabilized the spinal segment (i.e. provided intersegmental control of the neck). The more lateral muscles acted as guy ropes supporting the vertebrae as they would the mast of a ship, and were more concerned with bending the neck (i.e. the control of neck orientation). It has been realized over succeeding years that the way in which muscles support and stabilize the spine is far more intricate than this simple model. Nevertheless, it is pertinent to address this issue of local (central) and global (guy ropes) muscles systems towards understanding muscle function in relation to the stability of the spine.

Bergmark[33] has categorized the trunk muscles into local and global muscle systems based on their main mechanical roles in stabilization (Box 2.1). The local muscle system includes deep muscles and the deep portions of some muscles which have their origin or insertion on the lumbar vertebrae. These muscles are capable of controlling the stiffness and intervertebral relationship of the spinal segments and the posture of the lumbar spine. The lumbar multifidus muscle, with its vertebrae to vertebrae

---

**Box 2.1**   Categorization of the lumbar and abdominal muscles based on their role in stabilization (after Bergmark[33])

| Local stabilizing system | Global stabilizing system |
| --- | --- |
| • Intertransversarii<br>• Interspinales<br>• Multifidus<br>• Longissimus thoracis pars lumborum<br>• Iliocostalis lumborum pars lumborum<br>• Quadratus lumborum, medial fibres<br>• Transversus abdominis<br>• Obliquus internus abdominis (fibre insertion into thoracolumbar fascia) | • Longissimus thoracis pars thoracis<br>• Iliocostalis lumborum pars thoracis<br>• Quadratus lumborum, lateral fibres<br>• Rectus abdominis<br>• Obliquus externus abdominis<br>• Obliquus internus abdominis |

---

attachments,[230] is a prime example of a muscle of the local system. An exception is the psoas major, the morphology of which, despite its origin on the lumbar vertebrae, indicates that it is designed to act exclusively on the hip.[40] In the abdominal group, Bergmark[33] suggests that the posterior fibres of the obliquus internus abdominis, which insert into the thoracolumbar fascia, form part of the local system. The significance of this insertion is uncertain, as Bogduk & Macintosh[38] found that the number of fibres arising from the thoracolumbar fascia varied considerably in their specimen sample and were absent entirely in some cases. The deepest muscle, the transversus abdominis, with its direct attachments to the lumbar vertebrae through the thoracolumbar fascia and the decussations with its opposite in the midline, can also be considered a local muscle of the abdominal muscle group.

The global muscle system encompasses the large, more superficial muscles of the trunk, and includes the obliquus internus abdominis and obliquus externus abdominis, the rectus abdominis, the lateral fibres of the quadratus lumborum and portions of the erector spinae (see Box 2.1). These muscles are not only involved in moving the spine, but are also responsible for transferring load directly between the thoracic cage and the pelvis. The main function of the global muscles is to balance the external loads applied to the trunk so that the residual forces transferred to the lumbar spine can be 'handled' by the local muscles.[33] In this way the large variations in external loads that occur with normal daily function are accommodated by the global muscles so that the resulting load on the lumbar spine and its segments is continually minimized. Variations in load are thus kept small and manageable for the local system. In recent years there has been a focus on the local muscle system in studies concerned with aetiological factors in chronic low back pain.

## The functional significance of the local muscle system

The function of the local, deep muscles of the lumbar spine in stabilization has been highlighted in Panjabi's[262,263] hypothesis of clinical instability, which emphasizes the concept of control of neutral zone motion. Anatomically, the deep muscles of the local system are capable of making a major contribution to spinal stability, being closer to the centre of rotation of the spinal segments and, with their shorter muscle lengths, they are ideal for controlling intersegmental motion.[265] The deep muscles of the lumbar spine have varying architecture for their control of segmental movement. The smaller intersegmental muscles, such as the intertransversarii and interspinales, may not predominate as mechanical stabilizers but have a proprioceptive role instead.[37,68] Overlapping multisegmental muscles linking adjacent lumbar vertebrae and the sacrum, such as the lumbar multifidus, have the capacity to, and have been shown to be efficient in stabilizing the spinal segment.[68] Additional evidence suggests that transversus abdominis also contributes to this function of segmental stability (see Ch. 4)

Further progress in understanding the aetiology of low back pain and the vital role of the local muscles in spinal stabilization has also come from the biomechanical study by Cholewicki & McGill.[54] In an attempt to quantify the mechanical stability of the spine during various functional tasks, they developed a biomechanical in vivo model (electromyography assisted). The model incorporated anatomical analysis, calculation of external loads, passive tissue forces and muscle forces. Notably, the influence of muscle stiffness, a critical component of the stability function of muscles, was included in the model. The results and conclusions drawn from this study confirmed the proposed relationship between the local and global stabilizing systems.[33] While the large muscles linking the pelvis to the rib cage provided a significant amount of stiffness to the spinal column, activity of the local muscle system, which crosses one or more spinal segments, was found to be vital in providing stability of the spinal segments. Even when forces generated by the large global muscles were substantial, the spine was unstable if there was no activity in the local muscle system. A small increase in the level of activity of the muscles of the local system could prevent spinal instability.

Cholewicki & McGill[54] considered that their model supported the hypothesis of the neutral zone and spinal stability.[262,263] Increases in aberrant or uncontrolled neutral zone motion could be countered by increases in activity of the local muscle system. These muscles, they believe, could be dysfunctional in back pain patients. The local muscles may not be able to maintain prolonged or sustained muscle contraction in order to protect continuously any unstable spinal segments, which could leave the low back pain patient vulnerable to persistent strain and pain. Other authors agree. Marras & Mirka[234] recognized that, while larger postural (global) muscles have a significant trunk-supporting role, the smaller muscles surrounding the spine are likely to make an important contribution to stability during 'motor generation and trunk control'.

Many of the traditional studies investigating spinal injury and back pain have modelled the situation where tissue tolerance has been exceeded in high-demand activities such as heavy lifting. Cholewicki & McGill's[54] model not only highlighted the prime role of local muscles in spinal stabilization at high loads, it also pointed to the importance of the local system in providing spinal support during low-load activities requiring only low muscle forces. Light tasks, such as reaching or moving while sitting or standing, do not require or recruit a large contribution from the strong global muscles. Nevertheless, the muscles of the local system are needed for safe function at the segmental level. Persons with or without a history of low back pain who may lack control of their deep local muscles could have poor segmental support during light activities (see Ch. 7). The authors proposed that repeated microtrauma to the same tissues over time due to a lack of deep muscle control will eventually lead to sufficient damage to trigger nociceptors and lead to low back pain. This proposal fits well with the clinical histories heard from many low back pain patients, and could be an explanation of how back injury could be precipitated or perpetuated by light functional activities. It also has significant implications for those interested in preventing first time or recurrent low back injuries.

## Limitations of the global system in supporting the spinal segment

While there is no doubt that the large global muscles surrounding the spine are vital to trunk postural and spinal support and control, the global system has limitations in providing spinal segmental support. This can provide a further indirect argument for the importance of the local muscles and for their rehabilitation in the low back pain patient.

### Control of shear forces

It appears that it may be in controlling shear forces at the spinal segment that the global muscle system has its severest limitations. In a biomechanical study of the back extensors, Macintosh et al[229] demonstrated that small changes in flexion of the trunk resulted in large changes in shear forces at the lumbar spine. Their study did not address the issue of which

muscles were likely to help counteract such shear forces. In an attempt to understand the way in which the trunk muscles control shear loading, Raschke & Chaffin[275] studied muscle recruitment in the lumbopelvic muscles (erector spinae, latissimus dorsi, obliquus externus abdominis, rectus abdominis, gluteus maximus and rectus femoris) using surface electromyography. These global muscles did not respond to induced shear loading of the spine. The authors believe that it is likely that the muscles of the deeper local system, which could not be measured using surface electromyography, were actively supporting the spine during such spinal loading.

A similar situation may exist in the sacro-iliac joints. Snijders et al,[312] from their work on biomechanical modelling of the sacro-iliac joints, describe how muscles, combined with ligaments and fascia, are used to protect the sacro-iliac joints against shearing forces. The compression force required to control shear forces is, to a large extent, provided by the large global muscles working in discrete synergies (e.g. the contraction of gluteus maximus with the diagonally opposed latissimus dorsi).[345,346] However, there is another system that is also operating to protect the sacro-iliac joints from shear loading.[312] This is provided by the architecture of the pelvis combined with the action of deep local muscles. The horizontal forces produced by the transversus abdominis and obliquus internus abdominis across the iliac crests compress and stabilize the sacro-iliac joints. The pelvic arch mechanism is also dependent on the action of the coccygeus and piriformis, in addition to the sacrotuberous and sacrospinal ligaments. The significant contribution of parts of the erector spinae muscles attached to the sacrum (e.g. the lumbar multifidus) is also recognized in this model. Thus the deep local muscles play an important role in the stabilization of the sacro-iliac joints. Of particular interest will be future studies that address the relative contribution of the local and global muscle systems in the protection of the sacro-iliac joints in a variety of functional tasks.

*Excessive spinal loading*

The contribution of the muscles of the global system to lumbar segmental stability in everyday situations is also limited by potential problems associated with the amounts of muscle activity and co-contractions necessarily generated by these large postural muscle groups. These problems can include excessive loads on spinal structures from unnecessarily high muscle forces and an abnormal rigidity of the trunk from over co-contraction of too many or the incorrect muscles.[138,257,281] Increased levels of co-contraction of the global muscles of the trunk is associated with increased compression and spinal loading.[205,244,330] While increased co-contraction is expected during lifting activities and with increased trunk acceleration,[234] excessively high levels of co-contraction of the global muscles have been detected in patients who develop low back pain compared with normal pain-free subjects (W.S. Marras, personal communication, 1994). Excessive global muscle co-contraction during light functional tasks may even be indicative of inappropriate trunk muscle control in back pain patients.[138,257] These clinical findings support the hypothesis of Cholewicki et al,[56] who studied the stabilizing function of the trunk flexors and extensors around a neutral spine posture. Their hypothesis was that a dysfunction in the passive stabilizing system may be indicated by increased levels of trunk muscle co-activation. This hypothesis challenges many current exercise programmes for low back pain that incorporate high levels of trunk muscle co-activation. These may in fact exacerbate the patient's muscle problem.

*A challenge to spinal loading*

Actions of individual global muscles may actually challenge spinal support. For example, Bergmark[33] considers that muscles linking the pelvis to the lower limb (e.g. psoas major) and the pelvis to the upper limb (e.g. latissimus dorsi) fall into this category. Lumbar segmental stability must be maintained in spite of the action of these muscles in functional movement.

In a similar manner, Snijders et al[312] demonstrated that the rectus abdominis and iliopsoas produce unfavourable forces for the stability of the sacro-iliac joints. Any overactivity and tightness in any of these muscles in back pain patients[163] could pose a problem in the rehabilitation of lumbar segmental stability.

## CLINICAL APPLICATION

It is well recognized that the osseoligamentous spine is inherently unstable,[69] and that in vivo it requires a combination of muscle forces and muscle stiffness (with different combinations of muscles) to make it a secure and stable structure.[106] From anatomical and biomechanical studies some guidelines can be gained for the principles of management for enhancing the stabilizing role of the muscle system of the lumbopelvic region. Such principles can help in devising appropriate preventive and rehabilitative exercises for low back pain patients.

Basically, there are two broad approaches for improving the spinal-protection role of the muscles which can be gleaned from anatomical and biomechanical studies on lumbopelvic stabilization. The first utilizes the principle of minimizing forces applied to the lumbar spine during functional activities. The second is to ensure that the deep local muscle system is operating to stabilize the individual spinal segments.

## Minimizing forces applied to the lumbar spine

There are several different ways to minimize the forces applied to the lumbar spine during everyday and work-related activities. The study and practice of ergonomics has increased knowledge and helped to establish suitable working postures, lifting techniques and furniture design which are essential in decreasing joint forces potentially harmful to spinal structures. Although not specifically addressed here, the value in addressing ergonomic principles in protecting the spine from injury cannot be overstated.

The other principle involved in reducing forces placed on the lumbar spine deals with strength and endurance training of the global muscles to enhance their torque-producing role during high-level functions such as heavy lifting. If the global muscles can cope with the level of external load required by an individual in their everyday activity this will ensure that the forces transferred to the spine itself are kept to as low and as manageable a level as possible. These forces can then be handled by the local muscle system.

However, global muscle function can cause potentially harmful effects if there is overactivity in certain muscles of this system. Methods of treatment aimed at decreasing any unnecessary activity in these muscles will assist in minimizing harmful forces. Logically this could only be safely pursued if the protective function of the deep local muscles was being re-established at the same time.

## The presence of an operational deep local muscle system

It is possible that, even if the global muscle system is working appropriately, the local system may not be operating well enough to control intersegmental motion[106] (Fig. 2.3). A deficit in segmental control while global muscle activity was near maximal was uniquely captured in vivo in a lifting study done by Cholewicki & McGill.[53] Indirect evidence of an active global system operating with a poor local system may be gained from the study of patients with low back pain associated with spondylolysis and spondylolisthesis done by O'Sullivan et al.[257] Subjects in the control group who performed general strength training exercises, such as swimming, gym work and sit-ups, failed to show any decrease in symptoms or increase in functional ability with this work for the global muscles. This was in contrast to the reduction in low back pain and increase in functional ability demonstrated by the experimental group who trained their local muscle system. This study highlights the importance of specifically addressing the local muscle system as the other

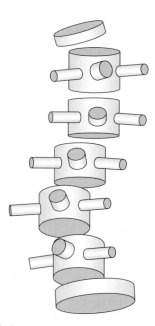

**Figure 2.3** A diagrammatic representation of a lack of spinal intersegmental control. (Adapted from Gardner-Morse et al[106].)

broad approach to enhancing muscular stabilization of the spine.

It has been realized from the more recent biomechanical studies that the local muscle system is important in providing support and control to the individual vertebral segments whether functional tasks are light (walking) or heavy (lifting) in nature. The picture emerging is of local muscles being required to contract continually, at low levels, no matter what functional activity is being undertaken. The functional supportive role of these muscles may not depend only on the development of force in the muscle, but also on the neuromuscular control and coordination of that force. Panjabi,[262,263] in his model of spinal stabilization, stresses that the neural control of these supporting muscles will be closely linked with development of appropriate tension. Poor stabilization will ensue if the forces developed are 'too small, too large, too early or too late'. Gardner-Morse et al[106] also acknowledge that, while various programmes for the prevention of injury and rehabilitation have been aimed at minimizing spinal forces, the possible 'destabilizing effects of poor neuro-muscular coordination' have not been taken into account. Thus the local muscle system and its control have been brought forward as possibly the most important factor in providing continuous spinal support. For these reasons it can be argued that specific testing and training of these muscles are required for patients with low back pain.

This line of thought regarding neuromuscular control and local muscle function encourages practitioners to particularly note the patient's mechanism of injury. The history of onset of low back pain may give the practitioner some insight into the origin of muscle problems as well as insight into the challenges likely to be faced in rehabilitation. Insidious onset low back pain or onset associated with a trivial incident is more likely to be linked to gradual tissue breakdown that has occurred over a period of time. The term coined by Gardner-Morse et al[106] for this type of back pain is 'self-injury', where the spine has not been adequately 'self-stabilized'. Inherent poor muscle control in the local muscle system, as well as decreased strength and endurance of the global system, could play a pivotal role in the development of such back pain over time.

The antithesis to this situation is one where direct overload to the muscles or substantial trauma to the spine has precipitated an acute injury. While this trauma would result in reflex muscle inhibition, inherent long-standing problems of the local and global system in their spinal supporting role may not be present in these patients.

## CONCLUSIONS

- A link can be established between dysfunction in the local muscle system and mechanical low back pain.
- The control of spinal stability is highly dependent on the muscle system, most particularly the deep local muscles of the lumbopelvic area.
- Segmental control by the deep local muscle system for spinal support has been linked to both high- and low-load functional activities.
- A problem in neuromuscular control of the local muscles by the nervous system has been suggested as one of the most important factors in the development or perpetuation of 'clinical instability' and symptoms of low back pain.

# 3

# Traditional views of the function of the muscles of the local stabilizing system of the spine

It is pertinent to review what has been studied in relation to the function of the individual muscles of the local stabilizing system of the spine. This will lay the foundation for new knowledge on the role of the transversus abdominis in the stability of the spine (see Ch. 4) as well as give an appreciation of the potential significance of dysfunction found clinically and in research in the lumbar multifidus and transversus abdominis in low back pain patients (see Ch. 5). Discussion of the muscles' function is preceded by a brief review of their anatomy.

## MUSCLES OF THE LUMBAR REGION

The muscles of the lumbar region that contribute to the local stabilizing system of the spine are:

- Intersegmental muscles:
  - intertransversarii
  - interspinales.
- Lumbar muscles:
  - lumbar multifidus
  - longissimus thoracis pars lumborum
  - iliocostalis lumborum pars lumborum.
- Quadratus lumborum (medial fibres).

## INTERSEGMENTAL MUSCLES

The *intertransversarii* and *interspinales* are small segmental muscles connecting the transverse processes and spinous processes, respectively, of two adjacent lumbar vertebrae.[37] Their small size and location close to the centre of rotation of the segment indicate that they would have little torque-producing capability. They have a segmental nerve supply,[41] and Bogduk[37] suggests that these muscles may have a predominant proprioceptive role. As such they could influence kinesthetic sense in the lumbar region and, therefore, affect patterns of muscle activity. At this time, it is not possible to undertake an evaluation of this functional role, and therefore detection of any impairment in their function in low back pain patients is, likewise, not possible.

## THE LUMBAR MUSCLES
### Anatomy

*Lumbar multifidus.* This is the most medial of the lumbar muscles, and of the three lumbar muscles has the unique arrangement of predominantly vertebra-to-vertebra attachments within the lumbar and between the lumbar and sacral vertebrae.[230] The muscle has five separate bands, each consisting of a series of fascicles which stem from spinous processes and laminae of the lumbar vertebrae (Fig 3.1a). In each band the deepest and shortest fascicle arises from the vertebral lamina. The lamina fibres insert into the mamillary processes of the vertebra two levels caudad with the L5 fibres inserting onto an area of the sacrum above the first dorsal sacral foramen. The other fascicles arise from the spinous process and are longer than the laminar fibres.[230] Each lumbar vertebra gives rise to one group of fascicles which overlap those of the other levels. The fascicles from a given spinous process insert onto mamillary processes of the lumbar or sacral vertebrae three, four or five levels inferiorly. The longest fascicles, from L1, L2 and L3, have some attachment to the posterior superior iliac spine (Fig. 3.1b). Some of the deepest multifidus fibres attach to the capsules of the zygapophyseal joints.[209,230] The lumbar zygapophyseal joints are covered by the multifidus on all sides, except ventrally where the joints are in direct contact with the ligamentum flavum.[209] The attachment of the lumbar multifidus to the zygapophyseal joint capsules

keeps the capsule taut and free from impingement between the articular cartilages.[209,230]

*Longissimus thoracis pars lumborum.* This lies lateral to the lumbar multifidus and consists of five fascicles which arise from the medial end of the transverse processes and connect the lumbar vertebrae to the ilium (Fig. 3.2). The fascicle from L5 inserts onto the medial aspect of the posterior inferior iliac spine, while the fascicles from L1–L4 form tendons at their caudal end which converge like a common tendon to form the lumbar intermuscular aponeurosis. This attaches to a narrow area on the ilium lateral to the insertion of the L5 fascicle.[37]

*Iliocostalis lumborum pars lumborum.* This is the most lateral of the lumbar back muscle group. It has four fascicles which arise from the tips of the transverse processes of L1–L4, and an area extending on to the middle layer of the thoracolumbar fascia.[37] The four fascicles insert onto the iliac crest, with the L4 fascicle deepest and the L1 fascicle most dorsal (Fig. 3.3). There is no

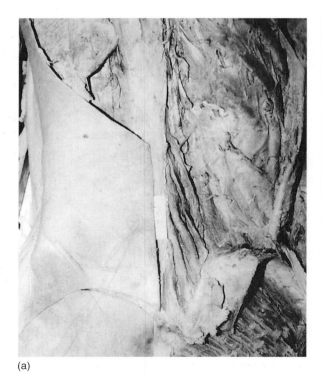

(a)

**Figure 3.1** The fascicles of the lumbar multifidus. (a) Anatomical dissection of the five fascicles.

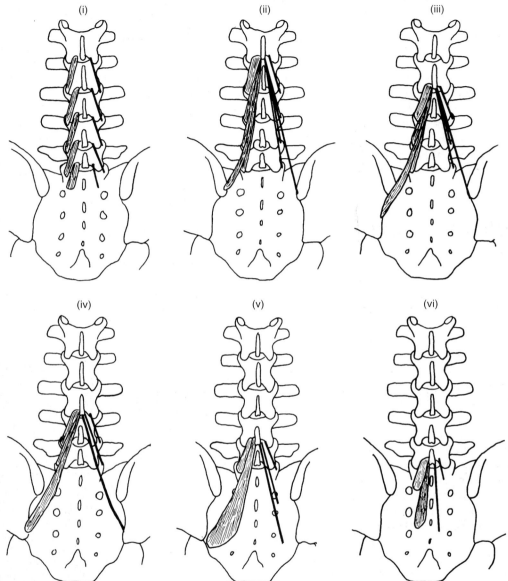

**Figure 3.1** (*Cont'd*) (b) i: the laminar fibres at every level; ii–vi: the longer fascicles from the caudal edge and tubercles of the spinous processes at levels L1–L5. (Reproduced with permission from Bogduk,[37] p. 106.)

muscle fascicle of the iliocostalis lumborum from L5 to the ilium in the adult. Any muscle fibres present at birth are replaced by collagen during growth and maturation to help form the iliolumbar ligament.[37]

## Function

The back muscles are primarily extensors of the spine when acting bilaterally, but the lumbar longissimus and iliocostalis can also assist in lateral flexion when acting unilaterally. None of

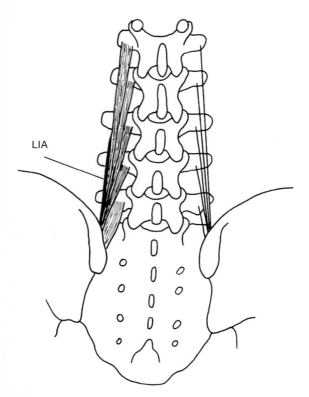

LIA

**Figure 3.2** Longissimus thoracis pars lumborum. (Reproduced with permission from Bogduk,[37] p. 109.)

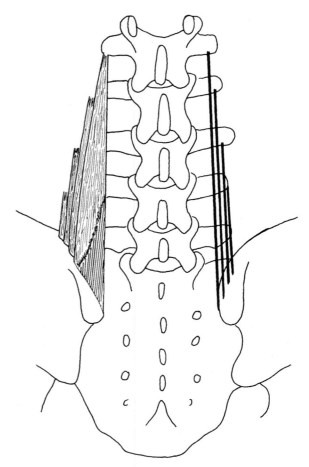

**Figure 3.3** Iliocostalis lumborum pars lumborum. (Reproduced with permission from Bogduk,[37] p. 111.)

the muscles are primary contributors to axial rotation, but activity in this movement may reflect their stabilizing counter to the flexion moment produced by the oblique abdominals.[37,227] In trunk flexion, the multifidus and lumbar longissimus and iliocostalis control the anterior rotation and anterior translation. On return to upright, the multifidus induces posterior sagittal rotation, assisted by the lumbar erector spinae which also control the posterior sagittal translation.[37] Nevertheless it is the thoracic components of the erector spinae which produce the majority of torque to extend the thoracic cage on the pelvis. The multifidus contributes only 20% of the total extensor moment calculated at the L4 and L5 vertebral levels; the lumbar erector spinae contributes 30%, while the thoracic components of the erector spinae contribute 50%.[39] Even though the multifidus is the largest muscle

at the lumbosacral junction, it is at a mechanical disadvantage to produce extension of the thoracic cage on the pelvis.

All three of the lumbar muscles contribute to the support and control of the orientation of the lumbar spine and the support or stabilization of the lumbar segments. The importance of their supporting function may be reflected in the distribution of muscle fibre type. In contrast to most human muscles, which have a relatively even type I and type II fibre distribution, several autopsy studies have revealed that the lumbar multifidus and the lumbar and thoracic components of the erector spinae muscles have a high proportion of type I fibres.[94,168,170,172,311,333]

These paravertebral muscles are also characterized by a large type I fibre cross-sectional area relative to other human extremity muscles and abdominal muscles (with the exception of the transversus abdominis).[170] The presence of both a larger percentage of type I fibres and a larger type I fibre size compared to type II fast twitch fibres supports the hypothesized tonic role of these muscles. The proportion of type I fibres in the thoracic erector spinae muscles has been reported to be as high as 70%,[311] while that in the lumbar erector spinae muscles varies in the range 58–69%.[94,170,239,311] When comparing the composition of the multifidus with the lumbar erector spinae muscles, a higher percentage of type I fibres, in the vicinity of 8–13% has been reported in the multifidus compared with the lumbar longissimus.[311,343] The exception was in the study by Jorgensen et al,[170] who found similar percentages of type I fibres in the multifidus and the lumbar longissimus.

The histochemical composition, capillarization and muscle enzyme activities of the lumbar multifidus and lumbar longissimus and iliocostalis muscles have been studied in vivo.[170] Multifidus muscle fibres have a large capillary network, with approximately four to five capillaries in contact with each muscle cell. The concentration of oxidative enzymes in all lumbar muscles is large and the endurance capacity high. This histochemical composition of the paravertebral muscles, with a high composition of type I fibres, indicates the tonic holding function, and thus supportive function, of these muscles.

Our particular concern with regard to the low back pain patient is the ability to rehabilitate the muscles that have the greatest potential to provide and substitute active support to the individual spinal segment which, from injury, has some passive insufficiency. What will be argued here, on the basis of morphological and biomechanical studies as well as studies monitoring the activity of the back muscles, is that the lumbar multifidus has better capabilities for segmental support and control and lesser capabilities for torque production. The lumbar longissimus and iliocostalis, on the other hand, have better capabilities for torque production and control of

spinal orientation but may not have as much specificity for function for one vertebral segment as does the lumbar multifidus. Furthermore, the more consistent activity of the lumbar multifidus in low-load functional activities may reflect its supporting function.

## Morphology

The unique segmental arrangement of the multifidus fascicles in the lumbar region indicates that it has the capacity for fine control of movements of individual lumbar vertebrae. This is reflected in its segmental innervation. Each fascicle of the lumbar multifidus and the zygapophyseal joint of that level is innervated by the medial branch of the dorsal ramus.[37,209,230] Each nerve innervates only the fascicles that arise from the spinous process or lamina of the vertebra with the same segmental number as the nerve,[230] illustrating the direct relationship between a particular segment and its multifidus muscle. This suggests that the segmental multifidus can adjust or control a particular segment to match the applied load.[23] The lumbar longissimus and iliocostalis do not show this tight segmental nerve–muscle relationship, suggesting a slightly more general relationship to the spinal segments. The lumbar longissimus is supplied by the intermediate branches of the L1–L4 dorsal rami, which form an intersegmental plexus in the muscle, although its fibres from L5 are innervated by the corresponding nerve.[41] The lumbar portion of iliocostalis is supplied by the lateral divisions of the L1–L4 dorsal rami, which run caudally, dorsally and laterally through the muscle.[41]

The cross-sectional anatomy of the lumbar spine is shown in Figure 3.4. What is of interest in the cross-sectional area of the lumbar back muscles is that multifidus muscle bulk increases on progression caudally from L2 to S1.[10,87] The multifidus is the largest muscle spanning the lumbosacral junction.[230] In contrast, the cross-sectional area of the lumbar longissimus and iliocostalis decreases on progression caudally. The large size of the multifidus muscle at the lumbosacral junction, when compared with the adjacent lumbar erector spinae muscles, also

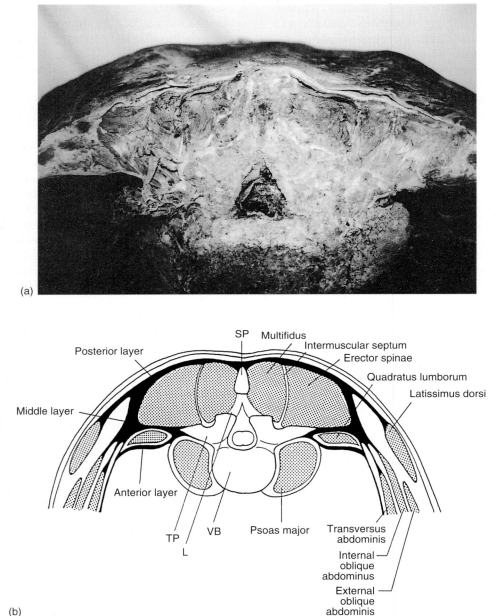

(a)

(b)

**Figure 3.4** Cross-sectional anatomy of the lumbar spine. (a) Cadaveric transverse section. (b) Schematic drawing of a transverse section showing the multifidus and the lumbar erector muscles (separated by an intermuscular septum), other muscles surrounding the spine and the layers of the thoracolumbar fascia (posterior, middle and anterior). L, lamina; SP, spinous process; TP, transverse process; VB, vertebral body. (Reproduced with permission from Porterfield & DeRosa,[273] p. 56.)

suggests that it is the muscle most capable of providing support at this level. Notably, it is the L4–L5 and L5–S1 segments that have the highest incidence of pathology in low back pain. The multifidus has a close relationship to the zygapophyseal joints,[230] and by controlling the sliding movement of the zygapophyseal joints in the craniocaudal direction it controls the distribution of stresses and loading on the vertebral triad. It is considered that the multifidus is the only muscle the primary function of which is to protect the vertebral triad.[209]

### Biomechanical factors

Several studies have investigated the lumbar muscles' capacity to increase the spinal segmental stiffness and, in particular, the control of neutral zone motion in line with Panjabi's[262,263] hypothesis of clinical instability. Studies have been done on various combinations of muscles to investigate their influence on these parameters. Kaigle et al[177] developed an in vivo animal model of lumbar segmental instability. Passive stabilizing structures (disc, zygapophyseal joints and ligaments) were transected and the effects of active musculature on spinal kinematics were examined in 33 pigs. Muscles surrounding the spine, including the multifidus, the lumbar portions of erector spinae, quadratus lumborum and psoas major and minor, were examined. The injured segments were subjected to muscle stimulation using wire electrodes. Results showed that increased, combined muscle activation stabilized the injured motion segment by reducing aberrant patterns of motion in the neutral zone.

Goel et al[110] used a combined finite-element and optimization approach to study the effects of the actions of the interspinales and intertransversarii, the lumbar multifidus and the quadratus lumborum. The introduction of muscle forces led to a decrease in displacements in the sagittal plane, anteroposterior translation and anterior rotation. It was shown that these muscles imparted stability to the ligamentous system. The load bearing of the zygapophyseal joints was found to increase, indicating that these joints play a significant role in transmitting loads in a normal intact spine. Muscle dysfunction (simulated by decreasing the computed force in the muscles) destabilized the motion segment. This led to a shift of loads to the disc and ligaments and decreased the role of the zygapophyseal joints in transmitting loads.[109]

Panjabi,[265] in an in vitro study of intact and sequentially injured fresh lumbar spinal units, again more specifically simulated the effect of intersegmental muscle forces on spinal instability. Simulated forces represented the multifidus (deep, shorter fascicles), interspinales and rotatores muscles. The segments were subjected to three-dimensional loads with increasing muscle forces. This study and the one by Goel et al[110] therefore examined the effect of the segmental muscles without the influence of the larger lumbar longissimus and iliocostalis. Panjabi et al[265] concluded from their results that the intersegmental nature of the deep multifidus fibres gave a tremendous advantage to the neuromuscular system for controlling the stability of the lumbar segment.

Wilke et al[354] investigated the influence of five different muscle groups on the monosegmental motion of the L4–L5 segment. The muscles examined were the multifidus (caudal and cranial directions), lumbar longissimus, lumbar iliocostalis and psoas major. Seven human lumbosacral spines were tested on a spine tester that allowed simulation of muscle forces. The combined muscle action of the muscles tested was found to decrease the total range of motion and neutral zone motion of the L4–L5 segment. The total neutral zone motion in flexion and extension was decreased by 83%. In lateral flexion, the total range of motion was decreased by 55% and the neutral zone by 76%. Under axial rotation the total range was reduced by 35%, but there was no significant change in neutral zone motion. Muscle forces were found to stiffen the motion segment. The strongest influence was created by the lumbar multifidus, which was responsible for more than two-thirds of the increase in segmental stiffness. The multifidus action was responsible for a significant decrease in the range of motion of all movements except rotation. These results supported those obtained by Steffen et al,[317] who in another in vitro study also found that the influence of lumbar multifidus decreased the neutral zone in flexion and extension.

The lateral stabilizing potential of the lumbar intersegmental and polysegmental muscles has also been investigated by Crisco & Panjabi.[68] They found that the polysegmental fascicles of multifidus and lumbar longissimus and iliocostalis fascicles were more efficient in this direction than were the short deep multifidus fascicles and intertransversarii and interspinales muscles. It can be surmised that the role of the multifidus in lumbar spine stabilization is complex. The multifidus is capable of controlling the neutral zone in the sagittal plane with its deeper, intersegmental fibres, but requires the assistance of the lumbar longissimus and iliocostalis in the lumbar muscles' contribution to the control of neutral zone motion in the frontal plane.

The deep multifidus fibres in particular are placed close to the centres of rotation of spinal movements and connect adjacent vertebrae at appropriate angles. McGill[219] confirmed the role of lumbar multifidus in a three-dimensional study of lumbar spine mechanics, and concluded that the unchanging geometry of the multifidus through a range of postures indicates that the purpose of this muscle is to finely adjust vertebrae with small movements rather than to function as a prime mover. The results of this study showed that the multifidus could function in this way in any physiological posture.

Muscles enhance spinal stability by increasing the stiffness of the spinal segment. It has already been shown that the multifidus acts to stiffen the motion segment.[354] From a mechanical perspective, the bending stiffness of the spine will also be influenced by other factors. One structure that can contribute to lumbar stabilization by increasing the bending stiffness of the spine is the thoracolumbar fascia. The thoracolumbar fascia constrains the radial expansion of the three lumbar back muscles.[23] It has been proposed that contraction of these muscles exerts a pushing force on the fascia.[91] The influence of the multifidus and the lumbar longissimus and ilicocostalis on the thoracolumbar fascia was investigated by Gracovetsky et al[117] using a mathematical model.

It was proposed that, because the thoracolumbar fascia surrounded the back muscles, it could serve to brace these muscles. The authors called this the 'hydraulic amplifier mechanism'. These forces may result in increased lumbar spine stiffness and contribute to lumbar stabilization.

### Control of shear forces

Shear forces are those that cause two vertebrae to slide with respect to one another.[37] During flexion of the lumbar spine, a forward or anterior shear is exerted on the intervertebral joint. Particular attention has been given to these shear forces, which are induced by bending and lifting tasks.[55,273] The control of anterior shear forces is essential for the protection of the intervertebral joint, especially at the lower lumbar levels where these forces are greatest. This control is provided not only by the passive elements and articular configuration of the vertebral column, but also by the muscle system.

Traditionally, the lumbar extensor muscles have been assigned this role. When contracting bilaterally, the lumbar longissimus and the lumbar iliocostalis can draw their vertebra of origin posteriorly, and hence oppose the anterior shear. On the other hand, contraction of the multifidus fascicles produces posterior sagittal rotation of the vertebra of origin rather than posterior translation. It is likely that during activities such as forward bending and lifting the induced forces are controlled by the lumbar erector spinae muscles and the multifidus together.

However, the control of shear forces appears to be a far more complex issue. A model of back muscles which mapped the actions of individual fascicles[40] showed that on maximal exertion shear forces can be induced by these muscles. From L1 to L4 the net result was a posterior shear force. However, at the L5 level the net balance was an anterior shear force. This would suggest that various muscles in addition to the back extensors may be involved in the control of anterior shear forces during lifting and bending tasks. Interestingly, Farfan[92] proposed that anterior shear forces were resisted more by the zygapophyseal joints, with countering forces in the reverse direction being provided by the abdominal musculature.

## The back muscles in posture and movement

It is possible that there are different primary functions for the different fascicles of multifidus. The longer fascicles, which originate from the spinous processes, have a mechanical advantage over the shorter, deeper fibres. The longer fascicles may contribute more to extensor torque, while the shorter deeper fibres, which have little leverage for torque production, may be more involved in a tonic stabilizing role. There is evidence to suggest this from electromyographic studies, where tonic activation of the deeper fibres has been examined during the maintenance of upright postures and during active trunk movements. Electromyographic analysis has allowed the function of the multifidus to be studied in vivo. Many classic studies have been performed using in-dwelling electrodes to access the activation of the deeper fascicles, which are likely to be involved in a stabilizing role. A tonic or almost continuous level of activation of the multifidus has been demonstrated in many of these studies of upright postures and primary active movements.

There is evidence that the multifidus muscle is continuously active in upright postures, compared with relaxed recumbent positions. Along with the lumbar longissimus and iliocostalis, the multifidus provides antigravity support to the spine with almost continuous activity.[20] In fact, the multifidus is probably active in all antigravity activity.[85,248,339] In the standing position, slight to moderate activity of the multifidus has been demonstrated,[85,169,339] exemplifying its tonic postural role. Furthermore, the multifidus is tonically active during walking.[248]

Results of studies performed in the sitting position have varied. It has been reported that the multifidus was inactive in relaxed sitting as well as when subjects were instructed to 'sit upright'.[339] In contrast, Donisch & Basmajian[85] reported that the multifidus was active in straight unsupported sitting, in accordance with its proposed tonic antigravity function. The differ-

ence in results between the two studies may relate to the way in which subjects assumed an upright sitting posture, and this becomes an important point in the clinical re-education of upright postural position.

Activation of the multifidus has been examined in forward trunk flexion and extension from the flexed position, trunk extension in the prone position and trunk rotation. An argument can be presented that the function of this activity appears to include primarily one of stabilization. As the spine bends forward from the standing position, there is an increase in multifidus activity.[97,248,270,339] At a certain point during flexion, the activity of the back muscles ceases; this is known as the 'critical point'.[97,185,186,248] It has been demonstrated that the electromyographic activity of the lumbar erector spinae ceases at about 90% of lumbar spine flexion. The critical point for the multifidus is not such a characteristic feature as it is for the erector spinae muscles. Although a decrease in activity is evident, in contrast to electromyograms of the lumbar longissimus and iliocostalis, those of the multifidus show silence infrequently.[339]

Extension of the trunk from the flexed position predictably evokes high levels of multifidus activity.[85,97,248,270] Marked activity of the multifidus also occurs when the trunk is extended or hyperextended in the prone position.[85,169,270,339] Even though, as has been mentioned, activity in the multifidus is marked in extension, the majority of the actual trunk extension torque (80% at the L4 and L5 vertebral levels) is provided by the thoracic components of the erector spinae muscles.[39] The multifidus has been shown to be active bilaterally in both ipsilateral and contralateral rotation of the trunk in sitting and standing.[85,169,248,270] For this reason, it has been suggested that, during rotation, the multifidus acts as a stabilizer rather than as a prime mover.[339]

As a general observation in movement studies, Donisch & Basmajian[85] reported that activity of the multifidus was related to its proposed action for only 50% of the time. Pauly[270] also showed almost continuous activity during the majority of the different directional activities tested. These findings can be interpreted as evidence for a stabilizing role of the multifidus rather than a primary role in torque production only.

## Summary

The lumbar multifidus, lumbar longissimus and iliocostalis play an important role in lumbar spine stability. Due to its unique morphology and segmental innervation, the multifidus would appear to be a muscle well suited to this role of segmental support and control. Biomechanical research has confirmed this important role. The biomechanical study by Wilke et al,[354] which included both the multifidus and the erector spinae muscles in the model, found that the multifidus had the strongest influence on lumbar segmental stability. The morphology of the multifidus, our clinical findings of a dysfunction in the segmental multifidus,[139] and later work such as that by Wilke et al[354] provide a basis for focusing specifically on the lumbar multifidus in low back pain patients.

## QUADRATUS LUMBORUM (MEDIAL FIBRES)

The quadratus lumborum consists of several laminae and is enclosed by the anterior and middle layers of the thoracolumbar fascia[37,355] (Fig. 3.4b). The medial portion of the muscle runs from the ilium to the anterior surface of the transverse processes of the lumbar vertebrae, and other fibres travel from the transverse processes to anchor onto the twelfth rib. The lateral portion of the muscle, which belongs to the global system, spans the lumbar area, attaching on the lateral ilium to insert into the twelfth rib without attachment to any vertebrae. The lateral fibres produce primarily a lateral bending moment. The medial portion, while unlikely to make a substantial contribution to lateral flexion,[37] is capable of providing segmental stability via its segmental attachments.[221]

Studies investigating the pattern of activation of the quadratus lumborum in functional tasks have been limited, because the depth of this muscle means that invasive electromyographic techniques are required.[12,221] In addition, needle insertion for fine-wire electromyography is both unpleasant and painful due to the thickness of the fascia surrounding the muscle (Hodges PW, Comerford M, Richardson CA, unpublished observations 1995). In two recent studies, which did use fine-wire electromyography, recordings were made from a midportion of the muscle, but there was no clear indication of whether activity was recorded from the lateral or medial portion of the muscle. McGill et al[221] provided evidence that the quadratus lumborum plays a significant role in the stability of the spine. Muscle activity was measured during a symmetrical bucket-holding task. Activity increased with increasing spinal compression provided through progressive axial loading. Further evidence for the general stabilizing role of the quadratus lumborum was provided by Andersson et al,[12] who found that, unlike the erector spinae,[185] there was no electrical silence of the muscle in full forward flexion.

While the results of these two studies support the thesis for a stabilizing role for the quadratus lumborum, we regard this muscle as a global stabilizing muscle, capable of controlling the external loads placed on the spine. Interestingly, in back pain patients, overactivity, tightness and trigger points are often reported by clinicians.[163,335] Treatment is focused on decreasing activity in the quadratus lumborum rather than increasing it with exercise. The medial portion of the quadratus lumborum may in the future be shown to be functionally separate to the lateral part of the muscle and contribute directly to the segmental support of the spine.

## MUSCLES OF THE ABDOMINAL WALL

The muscles of the abdominal wall that contribute to the local stabilizing system of the spine are:

- Transversus abdominis
- Obliquus internus abdominis.

## TRANSVERSUS ABDOMINIS

### Anatomy

The transversus abdominis, the deepest of the abdominal muscles, arises from the thoraco-lumbar fascia between the iliac crest and the twelfth rib at the lateral raphe, the internal aspects of the lower six costal cartilages, where it interdigitates with the diaphragm, the lateral third of the inguinal ligament and the anterior two-thirds of the inner lip of the iliac crest (Fig. 3.5). The medial attachment of the muscle is a complex and variable bilaminar aponeurosis. The lower fibres arise from the inguinal ligament and pass down and medially, blending with fibres of the obliquus internus abdominis to form the conjoint tendon, which attaches to the pubic crest behind the superficial inguinal ring. The remaining fibres pass transversely and medially to the midline, where they decussate and blend with the linea alba.[155,355] Above the umbilicus, the aponeurotic fibres of transversus abdominis pass either upward or downward and pass posterior to the rectus abdominis

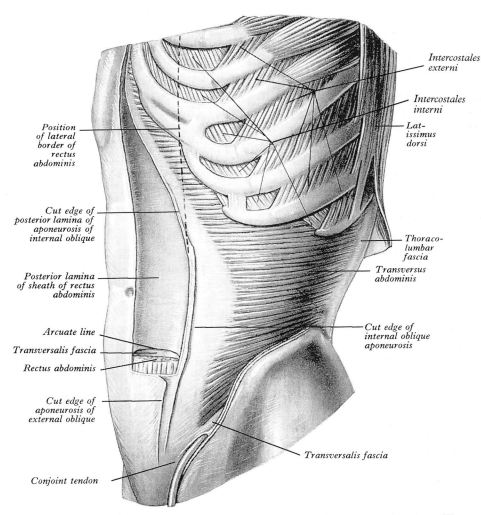

**Figure 3.5**  The transversus abdominis. (Reproduced with permission from Williams et al,[355] p. 599.)

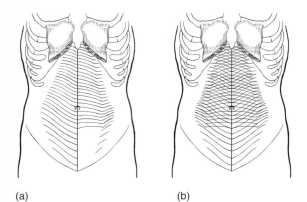

(a)                                        (b)

**Figure 3.6** The transversus abdominis anterior attachment. There are two layers of the aponeurosis. (a) The superomedial fibres on the right are continuous with the inferomedial fibres on the left. (b) The completed pattern of the two layers. (Adapted from Askar,[19] p. 318.)

(Fig. 3.6). The down-turned fibres attach to the upturned fibres of the opposite transversus abdominis or the posterior lamina of the contralateral obliquus internus abdominis aponeurosis. In contrast, below the umbilicus both layers are inclined downwards, with the anterior portion passing in front of the rectus abdominis and the posterior portion passing behind.[19,287] Proceeding from the umbilicus to the pubic crest, the fibres of the posterior layer are progressively transferred to pass anterior to the rectus abdominis.[287] Due to the decussation in the midline, the transversus abdominis can be considered to be a digastric muscle, attaching to either the contralateral transversus abdominis or the obliquus internus abdominis.[19,287]

The posterior attachment of the transversus abdominis to the lumbar vertebrae is via the thoracolumbar fascia. The thoracolumbar fascia is composed of three layers that are fused at the lateral border of the erector spinae, i.e. the lateral raphe. The anterior layer arises from the anterior surface of the transverse process of the lumbar vertebrae and passes as a thin fibrous layer over the anterior surface of quadratus lumborum.[38] The middle layer is a thick strong aponeurotic structure passing transversely from the length and tips of the lumbar transverse processes and intertransverse

ligaments in a divergent manner.[329] The fibres arising from L1–L2 attach to the twelfth rib, while those fibres below this level and extending to the iliac crest give rise to the transversus abdominis (the origin of the obliquus internus abdominis is variable).[38] The superficial fibres of the middle layer attach to the deep lamina of posterior layer at the lateral raphe, forming the sheath around the erector spinae muscles.[329]

The posterior layer is composed of two clearly defined laminae, which attach to the thoracic and lumbar spinous processes and the interspinous and supraspinous ligaments[38,329] (Fig. 3.7). The superficial lamina has a caudomedial orientation, forming the aponeurosis of latissimus dorsi and serratus posterior inferior, consisting of four main portions: the lowest group of fibres attaches by short fibres to the iliac crest; moving medially, the next fibres are angled at 20–30° below horizontal attaching to the L5 and sacral levels; the third group is deflected medially at the lateral border of erector spinae to 20–30° below horizontal, attaching to L3–L5; and the final portion covers the erector spinae.[38] Some fibres of the superficial lamina also attach to the gluteus maximus and obliquus externus abdominis.[345] Below L4, the fibres cross to the contralateral side and attach to the sacrum, iliac crest and posterior superior iliac spine.[345]

In contrast, the deep lamina of the posterior layer has a caudolateral orientation passing from the spinous process and interspinous ligament at a 20–30° angle below horizontal. The fibres from L4–S1 attach directly to the iliac crest and the posterior superior iliac spine. Above this level the deep lamina covers the erector spinae muscles, attaching to the middle layer at the lateral raphe. The fibres arising from T12–L2 are sparse and angled at 15–40° below the horizontal. The fibres of the deep lamina are fused with those of the superficial lamina in the sacral region and are continuous with the sacrotuberous ligament.[345]

The transversus abdominis is innervated by the anterior primary rami of the lower six thoracic spinal nerves (T7–12) and first lumbar spinal nerve (L1).[155,355]

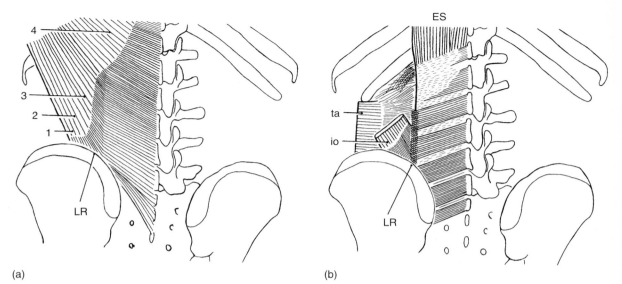

**Figure 3.7**   Thoracolumbar fascia. The superficial (a) and deep (b) lamina of the posterior layer. The superficial lamina can be divided into four major components, as described in the text. Both laminae have an extensive attachment to the lateral raphe (LR), which also serves as an attachment for the transversus abdominis (ta) and the obliquus internus abdominis (io). ES, erector spinae. (Reproduced with permission from Bogduk,[37] pp. 116–117.)

## Function

When the transversus abdominis contracts bilaterally it produces a drawing in of the abdominal wall, resulting in an increased pressure within the abdominal cavity[64] and an increase in tension in the thoracolumbar fascia.[329] As a result of these actions the transversus abdominis has been suggested to contribute to both supporting and torque-producing roles. These include control of the abdominal contents, contributions to respiration, the production of trunk extension (to maintain the stability of the spine against external forces causing the spine to flex) and the production of trunk rotation. Whether this muscle contracts unilaterally and what biomechanical effect such a contraction has, are subject to debate.

### Contribution to the support of the abdominal contents

One function attributed to the abdominal muscles is support of the abdominal contents. Due to the circumferential arrangement of transversus abdominis, this muscle is considered to have the most appropriate mechanical efficiency to perform this role.[83] Concurrently, activity of transversus abdominis[325] and the other abdominal muscles[48,49,96] is commonly reported in standing. However, this activity can be abolished easily with minor adjustment to posture or voluntary effort.[5,48,145] Changes in magnitude of activity with changes in position are consistent with the role of this activity in visceral support. The activity of transversus abdominis and the other abdominal muscles is absent in the supine position,[47,81,112] but increases as the head is tilted up to 45° or down to 45°, with greater activity in the dependent portion of the abdomen where the hydrostatic pressure exerted by the abdominal contents on the abdominal wall is greatest.[81] An additional benefit of this activity of the abdominal muscles is the reduction of the respiratory volume to below functional residual capacity.[81]

### Contribution to respiration

Electromyograms of the abdominal muscles recorded during quiet breathing show that these muscles are activated towards the end of expiration once ventilation has increased.[47,83,96,112,325] Contraction of the abdominal muscles contributes to the regulation of the length of the diaphragm,[81] end-expiratory lung volume[131] and expiratory airflow.[5] With voluntary increases in expiratory force (e.g. expiration below the functional residual capacity and forced expiration against a closed glottis), all the abdominal muscles contract in concert.[83,112] However, when the ventilation is increased involuntarily, by rebreathing $CO_2$ or with provision of an inspiratory load, the transversus abdominis is recruited at lower levels of ventilation than the obliquus externus abdominis or rectus abdominis.[1,83,347] This contraction of the transversus abdominis results in increased inspiratory efficiency by increasing the length of the diaphragm, and permits elastic recoil of the thoracic cavity to contribute to the initiation of inspiration.[131,237]

*Contribution to production of intra-abdominal pressure*

Although each of the abdominal muscles may flatten the abdominal wall and compress the abdominal viscera,[178,355] the circumferential arrangement of the transversus abdominis allows this muscle to have the greatest efficiency in increasing intra-abdominal pressure (IAP).[83] This is particularly important when flexion of the trunk is to be avoided,[26] which would occur if the other flexing abdominal muscles were active. In agreement, several recent reports have identified a strong relationship (compared with the other abdominal muscles) between the electromyographic activity of the transversus abdominis and the IAP on isokinetic lifting and lowering,[67] trunk extension,[64] and inertial loading of trunk movement.[62]

*Contribution to trunk rotation*

Debate exists about whether a unilateral contraction of the transversus abdominis may produce axial trunk rotation. Although DeTroyer et al[83] reported little or no activity of the transversus abdominis with resisted rotation in sitting,

Cresswell et al[64] recorded activity of the transversus abdominis on the side rotated towards or bilateral activity, with the greatest activity in the ipsilateral side. Similar findings were obtained by Hemborg (personal communication, 1997) using surgically implanted fine-wire electromyography. However, recent studies have indicated that the activation of the transversus abdominis is not altered by changes in rotational demands in association with a postural perturbation produced by limb movement.[147,148]

It was suggested by Cresswell et al[64] that the contribution of the transversus abdominis to spinal stability may be its ability to control rotation produced by inequalities in the activation of the oblique abdominal muscles. In an additional study by Cresswell et al,[63] subjects underwent a training programme of resisted trunk rotation. At the end of training some changes in the rate of development of IAP were identified in functional tasks. What this change means functionally and whether it was due to changes in the transversus abdominis is as yet unclear.

The biomechanical mechanism through which the transversus abdominis may contribute to rotation is unclear, but it may relate to the decussation and attachment of the transversus abdominis to the contralateral obliquus internus abdominis, and to the oblique orientation of the aponeurotic layers of the medial attachment of transversus abdominis.[19,355] In addition, a recent study has proposed that the transversus abdominis may make a minor contribution to trunk flexion and rotation via its attachment on the linea semilunaris.[220] Finally, the transversus abdominis may not produce rotation but may restrict rotation or return the spine to neutral rotation from a rotated position by tensioning the lateral attachment of the thoracolumbar fascia (see Ch. 4). This issue has not been resolved.

*Contribution to control of trunk flexion loading*

One function of the transversus abdominis that has been discussed for many years, although not directly in relation to the transversus abdominis, is the possible contribution of increased IAP and

tension in the thoracolumbar fascia to the production of an extension movement of the
trunk.[90,116,121] More recent evidence suggests that
this may not be the case. It is important to
review this literature in order to provide a basis
for the contemporary views of the contribution
of the transversus abdominis to spinal stability,
as outlined in Chapter 4.

Observations of lumbar extension produced
by bilateral lateral tension of the thoracolumbar
fascia in cadavers[90] and theoretical evaluations
of thoracolumbar fascia anatomy[91] have led to
the proposal that the transversus abdominis could
produce an extensor torque due to the oblique
orientation of the fibres of the fascia. The tension
of the thoracolumbar fascia can be maintained
by contraction of the abdominal muscles.[92] The
transversus abdominis is likely to have the greatest
influence on the tension of the thoracolumbar
fascia due to its extensive attachment. The attachment of the transversus abdominis to the entire
lateral raphe allows this muscle to exert tension
on the middle and posterior layers of the thoracolumbar fascia in the middle and lower regions
of the fascia.[38] In contrast, the attachment of the
posterior fibres of the obliquus internus abdominis
is restricted to the portion of the lateral raphe
connected to the L3–L5 spinous processes.[38] When
the fibres of the obliquus internus abdominis are
tractioned, no visible displacement of the deep
lamina of the posterior layer is produced.[345]

It has been suggested that the orientation of
the fibres of the posterior layer of the thoracolumbar fascia may assist in the production of an
extensor moment by converting lateral tension
to longitudinal tension (Fig. 3.8)[116,117] At any
point along the lateral raphe there is a fibre of
the superficial lamina passing caudomedially
and a fibre of the deep lamina passing caudo-
laterally towards the spine, these forming a
series of triangles, each subtending two levels.[116]
Due to the obliquity of the attachment, the force
exerted at the basal angle would have a horizontal and a vertical vector. With bilateral tension,
the sum of the horizontal vectors is zero, while
the vertical vectors produce opposite movement
approximating the spinous processes (or preventing separation of the spinous processes) and

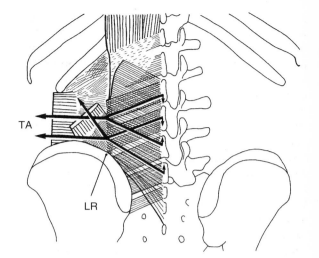

**Figure 3.8** The mechanics of the thoracolumbar fascia.
From any point in the lateral raphe (LR), lateral tension in the
posterior layer of thoracolumbar fascia is transmitted upwards
through the deep lamina of the posterior layer, and downwards
through the superficial layer. Because of the obliquity of these
lines of tension, a small downward vector is generated at the
midline attachment of the deep lamina, and a small upward
vector is generated at the midline attachment of the superficial
lamina. These mutually opposite vectors tend to approximate
or oppose the separation of the L2 and L4, and L3 and L5
spinous processes. Lateral tension on the fascia can be
exerted by the transversus abdominis (TA), and to a lesser
extent by the few fibres of the internal oblique muscle when
they attach to the lateral raphe. (Reproduced with permission
from Bogduk,[37] p. 123.)

resulting in trunk extension.[116,117] This provides
a mechanism for the transversus abdominis
contraction to contribute directly to extension.

Gracovetsky and colleagues[116] believed the
angulation of the fibres was in the range 12–60°
from the horizontal (depending on the angle of
trunk flexion), and calculated that the mechanism may produce a gain from lateral tension to
longitudinal tension of approximately 5 : 1, contributing significantly to trunk extension. Three
studies have since been done to evaluate this
theoretical model, and indicated a much less significant contribution.[223,228,329] Macintosh et al[228]
calculated the potential contribution of this
mechanism to extension production using data
derived from anatomical dissections, and identified
the true orientation of the fibres of the posterior
layer to be 30° to the horizontal (increasing to
40° with trunk flexion).[38] Assuming that the cross-

sectional area of the transversus abdominis is 2 mm × 70 mm, this mechanism could contribute 3.9 Nm to the extensor moment, or 5.9 Nm with the spine in full flexion. This contribution would be only 2% of the maximum extensor moment produced by the back muscles (i.e. 250–280 Nm).[115]

Furthermore, in a separate study, McGill & Norman[223] calculated the contribution of the tension in the thoracolumbar fascia to trunk extension to be negligible (less than 4%) compared with the force required to maintain a load in the hands. Tesh and colleagues[329] reported a gain of 0.42 for the conversion of lateral tension to longitudinal tension in full flexion with a fibre orientation of 15° to the horizontal. When tension of the thoracolumbar fascia was produced in a cadaver, no approximation of the spinous processes was observed. Clearly the potential for lateral tension of the thoracolumbar fascia produced by contraction of the abdominal muscles to produce spinal extension is minimal. A final concern regarding the contribution of the abdominal muscles to lumbar extension is the absence of attachment of the fibres of the thoracolumbar fascia originating from the abdominal muscles to the sacrum.[38] This makes it difficult to justify an extensor mechanism that is unable to transmit forces to the pelvis.[223] However, the small amount of compression produced by this mechanism may contribute to the control of shearing forces.

Alternatively, changes in IAP have been associated with control of spinal flexion forces. Early estimations of compressive loads on the spine resulting from trunk extensor muscle activity during lifting, identified loads in excess of the physiological limit of intervertebral discs.[26] On this basis it was concluded that an additional mechanism must contribute to the production of an extensor moment. It was considered that the abdominal cavity could function as a pressurized 'balloon' in front of the spine acting to separate the diaphragm and pelvic floor and thus produce a trunk extensor moment (Fig. 3.9).[26,121,248] Since this mechanism was considered to have a larger moment arm than the trunk extensor muscles, the resultant disc compression would be less.[26,332,337] It has been calculated mathematically that the load on the extensor muscles

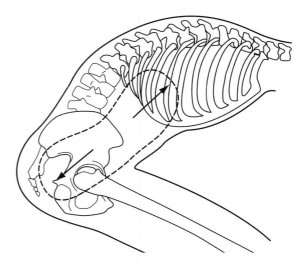

**Figure 3.9** The contribution of intra-abdominal pressure to the production of an extensor movement by exerting a distracting force between the diaphragm and pelvic floor. (Adapted from Bartelink,[26] p. 722.)

could be reduced by 12–20% as a result of this mechanism.[332] Consistent with this, a decrease in extensor muscle activity as a result of increased IAP has been reported.[226,349]

In support of this hypothesis, increased IAP has been associated with lifting, running and walking[26,121,199] and prior to jumping.[62,125] Furthermore, the magnitude of the IAP has been found to be linearly related to the magnitude of *static* flexion moments.[26,73–75,119,129,232,233,249] However, many studies of *dynamic* loading have failed to find a relationship.[233,302,337] Yet, a linear relationship has been identified in dynamic lifting and lowering.[67] Furthermore, increases in IAP are also associated with trunk extension loading, which is contradictory to the initial hypothesis.[119]

Several factors have been outlined in the literature that further question the trunk extensor role of the IAP; namely, the concurrent flexor torque produced by the rectus abdominis, obliquus externus abdominis and obliquus internus abdominis, the surface area of the diaphragm through which the abdominal pressure can act, and the magnitude of pressure required to produce an effective extensor moment.

Early mathematical evaluation of the potential trunk extensor moment produced by the development of IAP failed to include the concurrent flexion moment produced by the rectus abdominis, obliquus externus abdominis and obliquus internus abdominis.[332] Addition of the flexor moment to biomechanical models (as suggested by McGill et al[222] and Floyd & Silver[96]) has been shown to decrease the potential extensor moment produced by the pressurized abdominal cavity, thus increasing the requirement for extensor muscle activity to overcome the flexor torque, and resulting in an increase in spinal compression rather than a decrease.[29,197,222] Consistent with this, Nachemson et al[251] reported an increase in intradiscal pressure with increased IAP with a valsalva manoeuvre. However, the muscle pattern involved in the performance of a valsalva is different to that involved with trunk lifting,[121] thus bringing into question the relevance of this finding. In addition, the studies done by McGill & Norman[222] neglect the possible significant contribution of the transversus abdominis to the development of IAP. As the transversus abdominis does not have a trunk flexor moment, the compromise of the trunk extensor moment is likely to be reduced. The failure of trunk flexor training to increase the IAP production in lifting and valsalva manoeuvres provides further evidence that the contribution of the trunk-flexing abdominal muscles to IAP development is limited.[129]

The potential for IAP to produce trunk extension is further compromised when realistic values of the moment arm for the action of the abdominal pressure on the spine and surface area of the diaphragm (compared with previous studies, see McGill & Norman[222]) are used in biomechanical models.[222,224] When realistic estimates of these parameters are used, McGill and Norman calculated only a minor contribution of increased IAP to the production of trunk extension, even with the potential contradictory trunk flexion moment of the abdominal muscles removed from the analysis. This has been supported in vitro in a study that simulated the effect of IAP on the diaphragm and pelvic floor by using balloons inserted into the abdominal cavity of a cadaver; no significant extensor moment was observed.[329]

On theoretical grounds it has been calculated that in order to lift a 100-kg load, the IAP required would exceed 250 mmHg which, if sustained, would occlude the aorta and restrict blood flow to the viscera and lower limbs.[130] Furthermore, the maximum capacity of abdominal muscles is 60–50 psi (0.4–1.0 MPa),[93] which is insufficient to produce the level of hoop tension required to generate such pressure. Although pressures of up to 200 mmHg have been recorded,[249] the pressure rarely exceeds 100 mmHg in normal function.[77] High pressures can be sustained for brief periods, and have been reported in several studies.[26,76] The peak pressure is generally associated with the peak trunk acceleration at the initiation of trunk movement, suggesting that the IAP may be involved in the preparation for acceleration of the trunk.[23,129,225,233,336] A more recent study failed to find a relationship between the IAP and acceleration; however, in that study the IAP was developed in advance of torque production, and the period between the development of IAP and trunk torque production increased as the velocity increased.[235] This finding suggests that the IAP may act as a preparatory action to stiffen the spine prior to rapid trunk extension. However, a recent modelling study has suggested that large IAPs produced under high-force conditions, such as weight-lifting, may produce an extensor torque.[71]

In addition, we have evidence from recent studies investigating the control of the trunk against forces acting to challenge the spine resulting from limb movement, that the timing and magnitude of increase in the IAP is not consistent with the demand for control of trunk flexion and the activity of the abdominal muscles in all tasks.[144] From the evidence presented it is likely that the development of IAP may contribute to the production of a small extensor moment, although the magnitude of this remains to be established. Finally, a recent modelling study has re-evaluated the efficacy of the IAP mechanism on the basis of new measurements of factors such as the surface area of the diaphragm, and has indicated that an extensor moment can be developed even at low

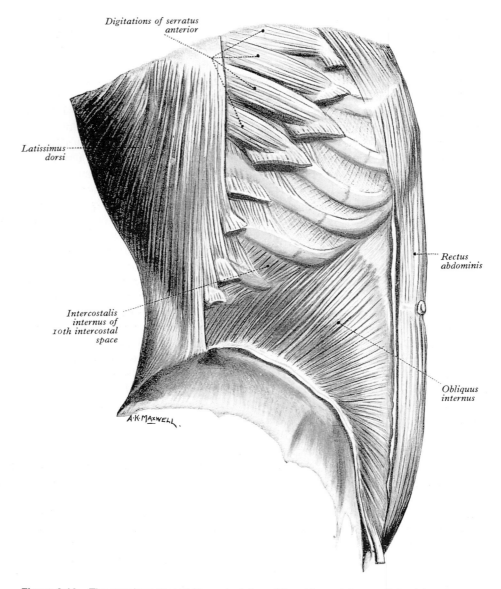

*Digitations of serratus anterior*

*Latissimus dorsi*

*Rectus abdominis*

*Intercostalis internus of 10th intercostal space*

*Obliquus internus*

A·K·MAXWELL.

**Figure 3.10** The attachments and fibre orientation of the obliquus internus abdominis. (Reproduced with permission from Williams et al,[355] p. 598.)

levels of pressure when pressurization is performed by transversly oriented muscle fibres (i.e. the transversus abdominis).[71] Thus debate continues regarding the extent of the contribution of this action of the transversus abdominis to the control of flexion moments.

## Summary

In summary, many functions have been attributed to the transversus abdominis. Although there has been much debate regarding the possible contributions of the IAP and thoracolumbar fascia tension to the control of trunk flexion loading, the evidence seems to suggest that this is unlikely to be significant. There is more recent evidence of other possible contributions of the transversus abdominis to spinal control, specifically to the control of spinal stiffness and intersegmental control. These aspects will be discussed in Chapter 4. Obviously, whatever the transversus abdominis does for spinal stability, this function must be integrated with the role of this muscle in respiration and support of the abdominal contents.

## OBLIQUUS INTERNUS ABDOMINIS

The obliquus internus abdominis forms the middle layer of the lateral abdominal wall, with a muscular attachment to the lateral two-thirds of the inguinal ligament, the anterior two-thirds of the iliac crest and the lateral raphe of the thoracolumbar fascia in a band 2–3 cm wide, attaching to fibres of the deep lamina arising from the L3 spinous process[38,355] (Fig. 3.10). The posterior iliac fibres pass superiorly to attach to the inferior border of the lower three or four ribs and are continuous with the internal intercostal muscles. The fibres from the inguinal ligament run inferomedially to attach to the pubic crest as the conjoint tendon with transversus abdominis. The intermediate fibres diverge from the origin, ending in a bilaminar aponeurosis with the upper fibres of the aponeurosis attaching to the outer surface of the seventh to ninth costal cartilages. The lower fibres of this intermediate region pass horizontally in parallel with the fibres of transversus abdominis.[155,355] The anterior layer of the obliquus internus abdominis aponeurosis passes superomedially towards the linea alba and lies anterior to the rectus abdominis. The position of the obliquus internus abdominis aponeurosis relative to that of obliquus externus abdominis varies depending on its position relative to the umbilicus.[287] The posterior layer of the fascia passes posterior to the rectus abdominis and has a similar arrangement to that of the transversus abdominis. The anterior fibres are continuous with the contralateral obliquus externus abdominis, while the posterior fibres are continuous with the transversus abdominis.[19,287] The innervation is identical to that of the transversus abdominis.

Similar to the transversus abdominis, the obliquus internus abdominis contributes to the support of the abdominal viscera and the production of IAP.[5] However, due to the fibre orientation this will be coupled with the production of a trunk flexion moment,[224,355] unless there is concurrent activation of the trunk extensors.[96] Cresswell et al[64] failed to find a consistent relationship between obliquus internus abdominis activity and IAP development. Due to the oblique fibre orientation, the obliquus internus abdominis produces ipsilateral rotation in conjunction with the contralateral obliquus externus abdominis.[64,269,355] Bilateral activity during rotation has been reported.[49] Bilateral contraction of the obliquus internus abdominis produces flexion of the spine[96,355] and contributes to fixation of the pelvis during leg movements.[96] Unilateral contraction results in lateral flexion.[49]

Although the obliquus internus abdominis has been generally categorized as a global muscle in relation to spinal stability, some portions of the muscle appear to function with the transversus abdominis in the local support of the lumbopelvic region. Bergmark[33] recognized that the posterior fibres of the obliquus internus abdominis inserting into the lateral raphe of the thoracolumbar fascia render this muscle capable of acting as part of the local support system of the lumbar spine. It shares this function with the transversus abdominis, which has a major attachment to the lumbar fascia. It should be noted, however, that this attachment to the thoracolumbar fascia is not present in all people[38] and thus may not contribute to segmental stability in these people. It may be speculated that the lower horizontal fibres of the obliquus internus abdominis could augment the action of the transversus abdominis in its role of supporting the sacro-iliac joints (see Ch. 2).

## CONCLUSIONS

A review of the muscles of the local stabilizing

system of the spine has determined that, of the lumbar muscles, the multifidus is that most closely linked to spinal segmental support. For the abdominal wall, the transversus abdominis emerges as a key local muscle. It is possible that some portion of the obliquus internus abdominis works with the transversus abdominis in its supporting function. Recognition of these key muscles, together with clinical findings in back pain patients, has helped focus our research on the status of the deep muscles of the local system in back pain patients.

# 4

# A new perspective on the stabilization role of the transversus abdominis

Although it has generally been accepted that the abdominal muscles may contribute to the stability of the trunk, the contribution of the transversus abdominis to this function has been largely ignored in the literature. This has been due primarily to difficulties in understanding how this muscle, with its transversely arranged muscle fibres, may contribute to spinal control. However, recent laboratory evidence has highlighted the specific contribution of this muscle to spinal stability and provided a basis for clinical observations.

Increasing evidence was arising from our clinical observations that changes in the function of transversus abdominis were present in people with low back pain (see Ch. 1). In addition to the clinical evidence, interest was developing in Sweden, where a research group headed by Cresswell was evaluating intra-abdominal pressure (IAP). They discovered that none of the superficial abdominal muscles could account for the IAP changes, leading them to evaluate the function of the transversus abdominis. Through the development of ultrasound-guided needle insertion techniques by Andersson et al,[11] DeTroyer et al[83] and Goldman,[112] it became practical to confidently record electromyograms from the transversus abdominis. Using this technique, two series of studies were begun: one by Cresswell, Thorstensson and colleagues at the Karolinska Institute, Stockholm; and one by ourselves.[140] These studies used both trunk movement and perturbations (challenges) to trunk stability to evaluate how the muscles of the trunk contribute to spinal control and whether the transversus abdominis was important in this mechanism.

In this chapter, the new evidence for the contribution of transversus abdominis to spinal stability is reviewed. This is followed by a discussion of the potential mechanism through which the transversus abdominis may contribute to stabilization of the spine.

## CONTRIBUTION OF THE TRANSVERSUS ABDOMINIS TO SPINAL STABILITY: NEW EVIDENCE

### Activation during static trunk efforts

In their initial experiment, Cresswell and colleagues[66] had identified an increase in IAP with both isometric flexion and extension of the trunk. Obviously this could not be accounted for by superficial abdominal muscle activity, since no activity was recorded in these muscles during trunk extension. This intriguing finding prompted these authors to evaluate the transversus abdominis in order to identify the muscle responsible for IAP generation. When trunk

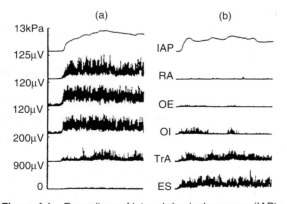

**Figure 4.1**  Recordings of intra-abdominal pressure (IAP) and abdominal (rectus abdominis (RA), obliquus externus abdominis (OE), obliquus internus abdominis (OI) and transversus abdominis (TrA)) and erector spinae (ES) electromyographic activity, showing activation of the TrA (and, to some extent, the OI) during both maximal isometric trunk flexion (a) and maximal isometric trunk extension (b) in a representative subject. Note the direction specific activation of the other abdominal muscles and the erector spinae. (Reproduced with permission from Cresswell et al,[64] p. 413.)

movements were repeated with fine-wire electromyographic recordings of the abdominal muscles, it was found that the transversus abdominis was active with both movement directions[64] (Fig. 4.1). Thus an explanation could be found for the IAP increase in trunk flexion and extension. But what was the explanation for the activity in this muscle? The authors proposed that transversus abdominis might be active to contribute to the stabilization of the lumbar spine either through the contribution to IAP generation or through the control of rotation. However, these results suggest only the function of transversus abdominis in a static situation. It was important to evaluate the response of the transversus abdominis with dynamic movement.

## Activation during trunk movements

In the next series of studies, Cresswell and colleagues investigated the response of the abdominal muscles in a dynamic situation.[64] In the first instance they evaluated movement of the trunk between flexion and extension in standing. On the basis of the previous investigation it was predicted that the transversus abdominis could be active with both movements. As expected, the flexing abdominal muscles, obliquus externus abdominis, obliquus internus abdominis and rectus abdominis, were found to be active in a phasic manner to contribute from the extension to the flexion phase of the movement. However, the transversus abdominis was active throughout the movement in both directions (Fig. 4.2). Once again the control of the transversus abdominis was related to the production of IAP, and the authors considered the results to suggest that the transversus abdominis may be contributing to stabilization of the lumbar spine.

Similar relationships between the IAP and transversus abdominis production and activation of the transversus abdominis, irrespective of movement direction, were identified with studies of lifting and lowering[67] and with movement of the trunk against inertial loading.[62] These studies evaluated both dynamic and static functions involving the trunk, and suggested that the transversus abdominis performs a unique function not shared by the other abdominal muscles.

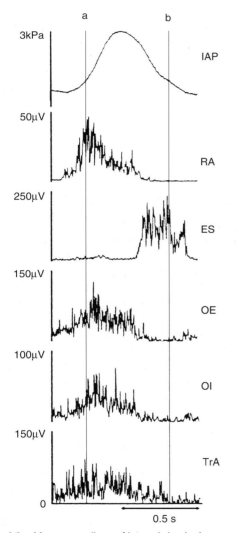

**Figure 4.2**  Mean recordings of intra-abdominal pressure (IAP) and abdominal (rectus abdominis (RA), obliquus externus abdominis (OE), obliquus internus abdominis (OI) and transversus abdominis (TrA)) and erector spinae (ES) electromyographic activity during four consecutive trunk oscillations between flexion and extension. Note the constant (but variable) activation of the TrA and the direction specific activation of the other trunk muscles. (Reproduced with permission from Cresswell et al,[64] p. 414.)

## Activation with trunk loading

Another means of evaluating the contribution of the trunk to spinal stability is to evaluate the response of the trunk muscles to perturbation. This method allows identification of the strategy used by the central nervous system (CNS) to protect the spine. Cresswell et al[65] chose to use this principle by adding a load to the trunk. A harness, to which a weight could be attached ventrally or dorsally to force the trunk into flexion or extension, respectively, was placed over the shoulder of subjects. When a load was added to the trunk to cause flexion forces, the authors identified a short-latency activation of the erector spinae muscles. However, before the erector spinae was active, the transversus

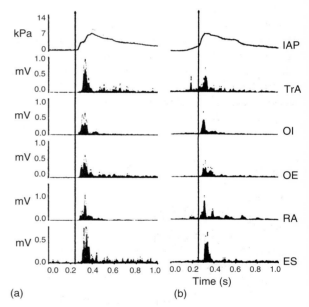

**Figure 4.3**  Rectified and smoothed electromyographic recordings of the abdominal (rectus abdominis (RA), obliquus externus abdominis (OE), obliquus internus abdominis (OI) and transversus abdominis (TrA)) and erector spinae (ES) muscles during unexpected front-loading (by the addition of a weight anteriorly to a harness placed over the shoulders) (a) and during self-initiated front-loading (b). The vertical lines indicate the onset of the perturbation. In (a) note the rapid onset of electromyographic activity of all muscles, with TrA being the first muscle to be active. In (b) the onset of activation of several of the muscles precedes the onset of the perturbation, although TrA is again the first muscle active, in a feedforward manner. (Reproduced with permission from Cresswell et al,[65] p. 339.)

abdominis was already active, with a latency of less than 30 ms (Fig. 4.3a). Similarly, with unexpected dorsal loading there was a short-latency activation of the flexing abdominal muscles, but once again the transversus abdominis was the first muscle to be active. The authors again proposed that the transversus abdominis may be functioning to stabilize the lumbar spine.

Cresswell et al added a final paradigm to this study. They allowed the subjects to release the weight that would load their trunk themselves. Thus, subjects had the ability to make predictions about the time and magnitude of the perturbation. When subjects did this, they chose to prepare themselves by initiating contraction of the trunk muscles prior to loading, yet the transversus abdominis was the first muscle active (Fig. 4.3b). The latency between the onset

of activity of the transversus abdominis and loading was approximately 100 ms, making it difficult to rule out voluntary preparation. Nevertheless, the results provide important information about the potential for pre-programmed activation of the transversus abdominis to prepare the spine for perturbation.

## Pre-programmed activation and limb movement

In order to determine whether pre-programmed activation of the transversus abdominis is an automatic component of the strategy used by the CNS to control spinal stability, it was necessary to identify an experimental model that removed the possibility of voluntary preparation. One such method of challenging the stability of the trunk is to move a limb. When a limb is moved,

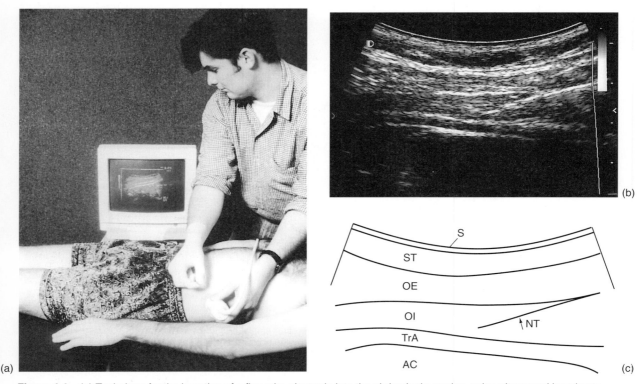

(a)

(b)

(c)

Figure 4.4    (a) Technique for the insertion of a fine-wire electrode into the abdominal muscles, using ultrasound imaging to guide electrode placement. (b) Ultrasound image of the abdominal wall demonstrating visualization of the needle tip. The muscle layers can be clearly identified by the bright white echo of the fascia separating the muscle layers. (c) The abdominal wall: S, skin; ST, subcutaneous tissue; OE, obliquus externus abdominis; OI, obliquus internus abdominis; TrA, transversus abdominis; AC, abdominal contents. In this case, the needle tip (NT) is located in the muscle belly of the OI.

reactive moments are imposed on the trunk, acting equal and opposite to those producing the movement.[42,158,363] With shoulder flexion, for example, the spine is caused to flex and rotate ipsilaterally as a result of inertial coupling between the segments.[42,144] In addition, there is a displacement of the centre of mass as a result of the reactive moments and the changed geometry of the body. Thus limb movement provides a method of challenging the stability of the spine in a way in which the CNS has exact information of when the perturbation will occur and how large the perturbation will be, as a result of years of movement practice. As early as 1967 Belen'kii et al[32] found that the electromyographic activity of the muscles of the leg changes in the period immediately preceding the onset of electromyographic activity of the muscle producing the movement. This pattern of leg muscle activity produces a postural response that begins before the movement, in order to

reduce the effect of the movement. The parameters of this feedforward postural muscle activity have been investigated in detail by many research groups.[42,59,100,158,363]

We predicted that if it is sufficiently important that trunk stability is controlled, then perhaps the CNS would activate one or several muscles of the trunk prior to the muscle responsible for limb movement. On the basis of the findings of Cresswell et al,[65] we predicted that the transversus abdominis would be involved in this response.

In our initial investigation we evaluated the abdominal muscles using fine-wire electromyography (EMG) electrodes inserted under the guidance of real-time ultrasound imaging[148] (Fig. 4.4). Subjects performed unilateral shoulder movement while recordings were taken from the opposite side of the trunk. As predicted, a feedforward response of the trunk muscles was identified. Furthermore, the transversus

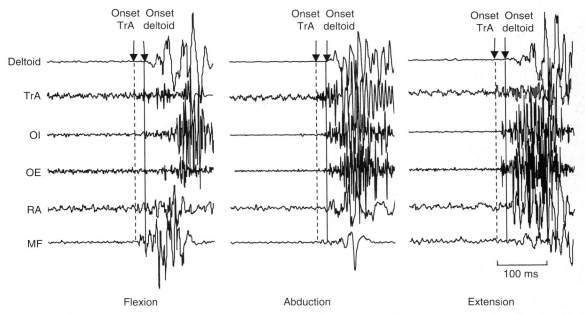

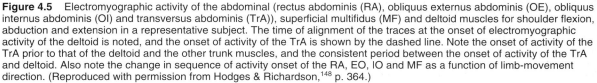

**Figure 4.5**    Electromyographic activity of the abdominal (rectus abdominis (RA), obliquus externus abdominis (OE), obliquus internus abdominis (OI) and transversus abdominis (TrA)), superficial multifidus (MF) and deltoid muscles for shoulder flexion, abduction and extension in a representative subject. The time of alignment of the traces at the onset of electromyographic activity of the deltoid is noted, and the onset of activity of the TrA is shown by the dashed line. Note the onset of activity of the TrA prior to that of the deltoid and the other trunk muscles, and the consistent period between the onset of activity of the TrA and deltoid. Also note the change in sequence of activity onset of the RA, EO, IO and MF as a function of limb-movement direction. (Reproduced with permission from Hodges & Richardson,[148] p. 364.)

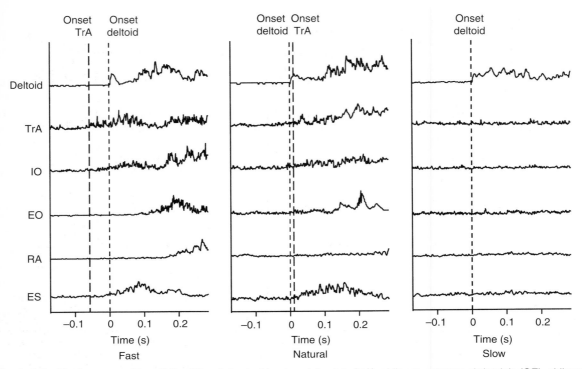

**Figure 4.6** Electromyographic activity of the abdominal (rectus abdominis (RA), obliquus externus abdominis (OE), obliquus internus abdominis (OI) and transversus abdominis (TrA)), superficial multifidus (MF) and deltoid muscles rectified and averaged over 10 repetitions of shoulder flexion at three different speeds of movement: fast (~ 300°/s), natural (~ 150°/s) and slow (~ 30°/s). The time of alignment of the traces is the onset of deltoid activity at zero; the onset of activity of the TrA is shown. The figure demonstrates the delay in the onset of activity of each of the trunk muscles relative to that of the deltoid with natural compared to fast movement, and the absence of trunk muscle activity with slow movement. ES, erector spinae. (Reproduced with permission from Hodges & Richardson,[149] p. 1224.)

abdominis was the first of the trunk muscles active, irrespective of the direction of the movement of the limb or the direction of the forces acting on the spine (Fig. 4.5). This finding provides further evidence that the transversus abdominis contributes to the control of spinal stability.

To confirm that the activation of the transversus abdominis is linked with the control of reactive moments produced by limb movement and not due to some other factor, two experiments were undertaken. In the first experiment subjects were requested to move their arm at different speeds: fast, natural and slow.[149] Since the reactive forces are dependent on the mass and acceleration of the limb, it was expected that with very slow movements the perturbation at the spine would be minimal. The results indi-

cated that the transversus abdominis was active in a feedforward manner with fast and natural movements but was not active with slow movements (Fig. 4.6). In the second study (P.W. Hodges and S.C. Gandevia, unpublished results, 1996), subjects performed movement of the shoulder, elbow, wrist and thumb. The transversus abdominis was active only with elbow and shoulder movement. These two findings indicate that the contraction of the transversus abdominis is dependent on the magnitude of the reactive forces, and that this feedforward activity is linked with the control of spinal stability.

In one further study we asked subjects to move a leg.[147] The leg is of larger mass than the arm and is in close proximity to the lumbar spine; therefore, greater forces would be transmitted to the spine with movement of this type.

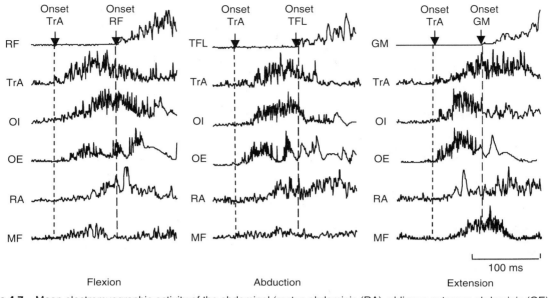

**Figure 4.7**    Mean electromyographic activity of the abdominal (rectus abdominis (RA), obliquus externus abdominis (OE), obliquus internus abdominis (OI) and transversus abdominis (TrA)), superficial multifidus (MF) muscles and the prime movers of hip flexion (rectus femoris (RF)), abduction (tensor fascia latae (TFL)) and extension (gluteus maximus (GM)) averaged over 10 repetitions for hip flexion, abduction and extension. The time of alignment of the traces at the onset of activity of the prime mover is noted, and the onset of activity of the TrA is shown. The figure demonstrates the onset of activity of the TrA prior to that of the prime mover and the other trunk muscles. (Reproduced with permission from Hodges & Richardson,[147] p. 139.)

Whereas the transversus abdominis was active approximately 30 ms before the prime mover of the shoulder, this period increased to 110 ms with leg movement (Fig. 4.7). This finding provides further support for the proposal that the transversus abdominis is active in the control of spinal stability.

## Activation with variation of the direction of the force acting on the spine

From basic biomechanics it can be expected that, when limb movement is performed in different directions, the direction of the forces acting on the spine will likewise vary. It was shown that the transversus abdominis was the first trunk muscle to become active with limb movement. It was important to determine whether this occurred with different directions of force acting on the spine. To test this we completed three electromyographic studies evaluating trunk muscle activity and trunk movement. In the first

study we confirmed that the onset of activity of the transversus abdominis was exactly the same with movement in each direction[148] (Fig. 4.8). In contrast, the onset of activity of the superficial muscles varied between movement directions. We interpreted this change in activity onset of the other trunk muscles as an attempt by the CNS to control the specific directions of the force. With shoulder flexion the early activation of the erector spinae was consistent with the requirement to control the reactive flexion movement expected to occur at the trunk. In shoulder extension, the early flexing abdominal activity of the rectus abdominis, obliquus externus abdominis and internus abdominis was consistent with the requirement to control the expected extending trunk reactive movement. These changes in the onset of activity of the superficial muscles are consistent with the findings of others.[17,100,363] The failure of the transversus abdominis to vary between movement directions provided initial insight into the possible contribution of this muscle to the

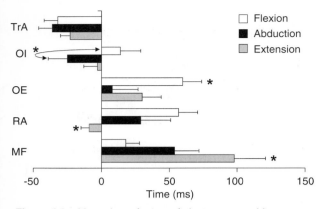

**Figure 4.8** Mean time of onset of electromyographic activity of the abdominal (rectus abdominis (RA), obliquus externus abdominis (OE), obliquus internus abdominis (OI) and transversus abdominis (TrA)) and superficial multifidus (MF) muscles relative to the onset of deltoid activity for all subjects (n = 15) for shoulder flexion, abduction and extension. All bars are aligned to the onset of deltoid activity at zero. The end of each bar indicates the group mean time of onset of the activity of the muscles of the trunk. Standard errors of the mean are indicated. Note the significantly different onsets in activity of OI, OE, RA and MF between movement directions and the non-significant variation in the latency between the onset of deltoid and TrA activities.* p < 0.05. (Reproduced with permission from Hodges & Richardson,[148] p. 365.)

generation of non-direction-specific stiffness of the spine with no direct contribution to the control of reactive forces. However, this needed to be confirmed by evaluating the magnitude of the electromyographic activity and spinal motion to confirm the direction of reactive motion of the spine.

In the second series of studies[142,144] we investigated the motion between segments of the trunk in three dimensions and electromyographic magnitude and timing parameters with unilateral and bilateral movement of the shoulders into flexion, abduction and extension. The results of this study confirmed the dependence of electromyographic magnitude and timing parameters of the superficial muscle on movement direction. In addition, the results showed once again a failure of the transversus abdominis to change in timing and also magnitude between movement directions. The movement analysis data also provided important insight into the strategy that the CNS uses to control spinal stability. The results confirmed

that shoulder flexion results in a flexion resultant motion at the spine and the converse with extension. However, prior to the onset of limb movement there is a small but consistent preparatory motion of the trunk in the opposite direction as a result of the superficial trunk muscle activity. This suggests that the CNS deals with the perturbation to the trunk by producing preparatory spinal motions, and not simple rigidification of the spine. This strategy has potential benefits for the absorption of forces by acting to dampen them. It appears that the transversus abdominis acts to stiffen the spine and maintain a stable intersegmental orientation in a preparatory manner in order to allow the action of the more superficial muscles to be simplified.

## Tonic activation

The pattern of response of the trunk muscles also provides support for the different roles played by the trunk muscles in spinal control. Ballistic limb movement is associated with a pattern of activation of agonist and antagonist muscles known as a triphasic response.[15] This pattern is typified by a biphasic burst of the agonist muscle separated by a single burst of the antagonist. Postural muscles are known to respond in a similar manner.[17,100]

It has been shown in several studies, including our own,[17,144,148] that the superficial muscles respond in short phasic bursts that are consistent with the preparatory and resultant spinal motions shown to accompany fast limb movement. However, in contrast to the other muscles, the transversus abdominis responds in a tonic manner in the majority of subjects. Generally, what is seen is a large initial burst of transversus abdominis activity preceding the prime mover, and then a longer duration, continuous, low-level tonic contraction. In a very recent study we have shown that the deep fibres of the multifidus respond in a similar tonic manner (P.W. Hodges, A.G. Cresswell and A. Thorstensson, unpublished data, 1997).

The tonic nature of the response of the transversus abdominis provides further indication of the supporting role of this muscle, and is consistent with both the continuous activation of transversus abdominis noted with repetitive trunk movement[65] and the function of other muscles, such as the vastus medialis obliquus with knee movement.[279]

## Independent control from other trunk muscles

From the evaluation of different directions of trunk movement[64] and limb movement,[147,148] it can be seen that transversus abdominis functions independently of the other trunk muscles. This separation in control by the CNS has important implications for the way in which we may approach the training of the transversus abdominis, and we required further investigation to evaluate more precisely the extent of this independent control. To do this we undertook a study in which the preparation for movement was varied.[152] The reasoning behind this study was that, since the pattern of response of the superficial trunk muscles is dependent on the direction of limb movement, the CNS would delay the onset of postural muscle contraction until the movement direction was known. In contrast, since the transversus abdominis acts in a similar manner no matter what movement is performed, it was predicted that the contraction of this muscle might not be altered if there is uncertainty about the exact movement to be performed. To vary the preparation for movement, subjects were told that they would be asked either to flex or to abduct their arm with varying amounts of certainty of the required movement direction. In some trials subjects were given a stimulus which told them the correct direction, in some trials they were given no information on which movement to expect, and in a final group of trials subjects thought that they were going to perform one movement but were then told to do the other.

The result of this manipulation of preparation was that subjects responded quickly when they knew what they were going to do, responded more slowly when they were given no warning, and more slowly still when they were given

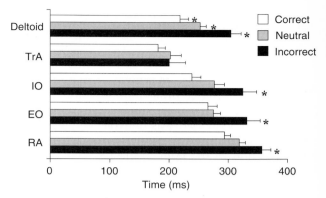

**Figure 4.9** Reaction time (mean and SEM) of the abdominal (rectus abdominis (RA), obliquus externus abdominis (OE), obliquus internus abdominis (OI) and transversus abdominis) (TrA)) and deltoid muscles from a visual stimulus to the onset of electromyographic activity of each muscle with varying levels of preparation for movement (correct, neutral and incorrect). It can be seen that the reaction times of all muscles except the TrA are increased as the level of preparation is decreased. This suggests a different control strategy for the TrA compared with the other abdominal muscles. *$p < 0.05$. (Adapted with permission from Hodges & Richardson.[150])

incorrect preparatory information. As predicted, when the reaction time for movement was delayed, the onset of activation of the superficial muscles was similarly delayed. This suggests that the CNS waited until it knew what movement to perform before it initiated contraction of the direction-specific postural muscles (Fig. 4.9). In contrast, the activation of the transversus abdominis was not influenced by changes in preparation and responded with the same reaction time in all conditions. In other words, the transversus abdominis was initiated as soon as the subjects knew they would move. Thus, the response of transversus abdominis appears to be a much more basic response with less information processing requirements than the other superficial muscles. This finding corroborates the earlier findings suggesting that a separate control system is used by the CNS to control contraction of the transversus abdominis.

## Activation and afferent input

The CNS can only make predictions about the expected outcome from limb movement in terms of forces acting on the spine. It was important to determine whether the simple early response of the transversus abdominis could be altered if the outcome from the movement was different from that which would normally be expected. To test this we performed an experiment where subjects moved the shoulder rapidly into flexion, as we had done before. However, in a small number of trials an external load was unexpectedly applied to the arm to cause a deceleration and further perturbation to the spine.[143] The results of this study confirmed that the pre-programmed response of transversus abdominis and the other trunk muscles is responsive to afferent feedback and can respond quickly (within 30 ms) after the onset of the perturbation to counter the challenge to spinal stability. This finding confirms that the transversus abdominis is responsive to afferent stimuli, indicating changes in stability requirement of the spine. It also provides evidence of a continually changing stability system of the spine.

## Contraction and mechanical response

All the trunk-movement and trunk-loading experiments undertaken by Cresswell and colleagues[62–65] measured a mechanical response of the transversus abdominis in the form of an increase in IAP, a necessary consequence of transversus abdominis activity. In addition, IAP changes were the most consistently related to activation of the transversus abdominis, as compared with other superficial muscles. However, it was uncertain whether the early transversus abdominis response identified with limb movement was sufficient to produce a mechanical response that could contribute to control of spinal stability. To assess this we undertook a study where the IAP and intrathoracic pressure were measured using a nasogastric tube attached with pressure-sensitive respiratory balloons.[145] When subjects performed rapid shoulder flexion, the pre-programmed early activity of the transversus abdominis was sufficient to produce an increased pressure in the abdomen that preceded the onset of limb movement (Fig. 4.10), thus strengthening the evidence for a contribution of

the transversus abdominis to spinal stability. However, the transversus abdominis is only one of the muscles surrounding the abdominal cavity. The diaphragm and pelvic floor muscles also contribute to the pressurization of the abdomen, forming the ceiling and floor of the abdominal capsule. Whether these muscles also contribute to postural control is an important question.

## The diaphragm and trunk stability

For many years scientists have searched for evidence suggesting a contribution of the diaphragm to postural control. These studies have involved the use of decerebrate animal preparations in an attempt to stimulate postural responses involving neck movements and simulation of thoracic afferents.[79,238] No such study has been successful in finding a response.

We evaluated the contribution of the diaphragm to postural control, using the limb movement model we had used previously.[141] In this study, the electromyographic activity of the diaphragm was measured using a monopolar needle electrode inserted into the costal diaphragm via the seventh intercostal space. A silver chloride coated band around a nasogastric tube (that also measures IAP and intra-thoracic pressure) was used to measure the electromyographic activity of the crural portion of the diaphragm transoesophageally. The activity of the transversus abdominis was also recorded. When subjects performed shoulder flexion, we found that both portions of the diaphragm contracted 30 ms prior to the deltoid (Fig. 4.10), i.e. at exactly the same time as contraction of the transversus abdominis. Importantly, this occurred during both inspiratory and expiratory phases of respiration.

The results provide evidence that the diaphragm does contribute to spinal control and may do so by assisting with pressurization and control of displacement of the abdominal contents, allowing the transversus abdominis to increase tension in the thoracolumbar fascia or to generate IAP. It is easy to see how this system

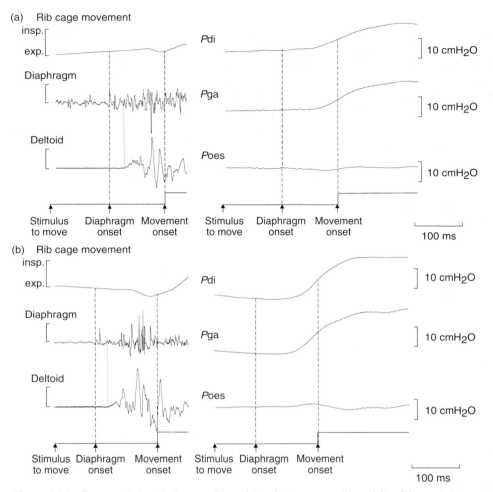

**Figure 4.10** Representative single recordings of the electromyographic activity of the costal diaphragm and deltoid, rib-cage motion, intra-abdominal pressure ($P_{ga}$), intrathoracic pressure ($P_{oes}$) and transdiaphragmatic pressure ($P_{di}$) with rapid shoulder flexion occurring during inspiration (a) and expiration (b). The onset of diaphragm activity and the initiation of movement of the limb are denoted by the dashed lines, and the onset of deltoid activity is denoted by the dotted line. The time-scale is identical in the left- and right-hand panels. The figure demonstrates the onset of increase in $P_{ga}$ and $P_{di}$ prior to the initiation of movement of the limb, thus providing evidence that the feedforward contraction of the TrA and the diaphragm is associated with a mechanical response that precedes the onset of movement. The figure also shows the onset of an increase in costal diaphragm activity prior to that of the deltoid, providing evidence of a contribution of the diaphragm to the preparatory spinal stability mechanism. (Reproduced with permission from Hodges et al,[141] p. 542.)

may function with short-duration postural tasks, but it is unknown how the diaphragm may contribute when the postural demand is sustained and the diaphragm must combine the roles of respiration and stability control. This is an area of ongoing research, but must involve eccentric/concentric phases of activation of the diaphragm. Several studies have investigated this function in patients who have undergone high spinal cord transection, and have provided supportive findings.[309,310] Recent evidence suggests that diaphragm activity may be associated with voluntary contraction of the transversus abdominis by drawing in the abdominal wall.[8]

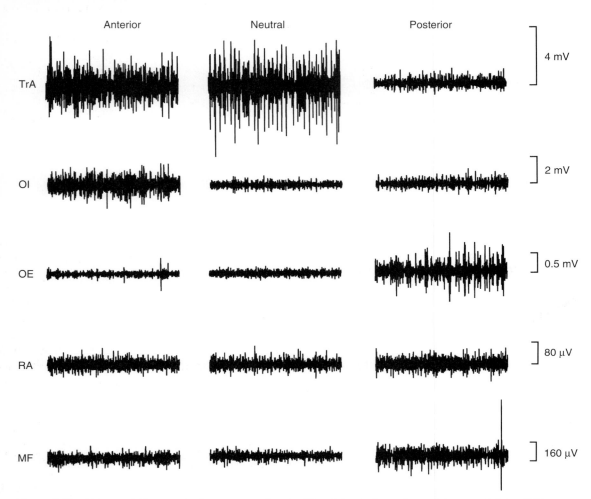

**Figure 4.11** Representative raw electromyogram of each of the abdominal muscles and the superficial multifidus during the performance of a submaximal pelvic floor contraction in supine crook lying. Contractions were performed in three conditions: anterior (anterior pelvic tilt with padding placed under the lumbar curve to maintain the position); neutral (with the spine and pelvis in a neutral position); posterior (posterior pelvic tilt with padding under the sacrum to maintain the position). Note the relatively isolated activity in the transversus abdominis with pelvic floor muscle contraction in the neutral position, and the additional activation of other abdominal muscles in the anterior and posterior conditions.

## The pelvic floor muscles and trunk stability

The muscles of the pelvic floor form the floor of the abdominal capsule and are an integral part of the muscular mechanism of abdominal pressurization. Preliminary investigations of the contribution of the pelvic floor muscles to the feedforward spinal stability mechanism have been undertaken. Results from EMG recordings of the pubococcygeus indicated similar onsets of activity as for the diaphragm and transversus abdominis (P.W. Hodges, C.A. Richardson and R.R. Sapsford, unpublished data, 1996). In addition, electromyographic studies done by Hemborg et al[130] have shown activation of the pelvic floor muscles in lifting tasks.

In two additional studies, we investigated the interaction between the muscles of the pelvic floor and the abdominal muscles.[298,299] In the first study, subjects were asked to perform maximal contractions of the pelvic floor while the electromyographic activity of the abdominal muscles was monitored using fine-wire electrodes.[298] When subjects performed the pelvic floor contractions, activation of the transversus abdominis increased significantly. In some subjects this was selective (Fig. 4.11), while in others there was also an increase in the activation of the other abdominal muscles. Interestingly, the contribution of the other abdominal muscles could be changed by changing the degree of the pelvic tilt and spinal curvature. In the converse experiment, the electromyographic activity of the pubococcygeus while abdominal muscle contractions were performed was investigated using fine-wire electrodes inserted through the vaginal wall.[299] Activation of the abdominal muscles resulted in an increased activation of pubococcygeus. Both of these investigations provide further evidence of a close neurophysiological association between these two muscles and suggest that similar centres in the CNS may be involved in the activation of these muscles.

## Respiration and spinal stability

Since the transversus abdominis is a respiratory muscle, there is potential conflict between the roles of this muscle in controlling expiration and spinal stability. It was important to evaluate how these two separate functions could occur concurrently. Previous investigations of the intercostal muscles provide evidence of modifications of postural activity on the basis of respiratory demand.[286] To evaluate this we asked subjects to move their arm at random points throughout the respiratory cycle and with different breathing conditions: quiet breathing, forced expiration and with inspiratory loading.[145] The latter two conditions were included because transversus abdominis normally only contributes to respiration when expiration is increased voluntarily by forcing expiration or involuntarily by breathing in against an inspiratory load.[83]

In relaxed breathing, no differences in the transversus abdominis onset timing were identified between phases of respiration (Fig. 4.12).

This finding suggests that the transversus abdominis can contribute equally well to spinal stability in any respiratory phase. However, when respiratory demand was increased, the transversus abdominis responded earlier in expiration than in inspiration (see Fig. 4.12). A similar change was noted for the rectus abdominis and obliquus externus abdominis.

There are two possible explanations for this finding. The first possibility relates to the influence of the respiratory drive to the abdominal muscles from the pontine and medullary respiratory centres. Although not yet shown in humans, there is evidence from cat research that respiratory motor neurons (including those of the abdominal muscles) are under the influence of a continuously varying level of excitability from a descending drive known as central respiratory drive potentials.[99,246,303] This descending drive causes expiratory motor neurons to be more excitable in expiration than inspiration. The earlier activation of the transversus abdominis with expiration could be explained by the increased excitability of its motor neuron pool in this respiratory phase.

Alternatively, the changes in timing may relate to the pre-existing levels of abdominal pressure. In inspiration, there is diaphragm descent and pressurization of the abdomen,[130] particularly when there is an inspiratory load. In contrast, during expiration the diaphragm is relaxed and abdominal pressure is low. Thus, during inspiration contraction of the transversus abdominis is required less and in expiration it is required more; hence the change in postural timing to accommodate this.

To test which hypothesis could explain our results, subjects performed a shoulder movement during the performance of a forced expiration against a closed glottis (valsalva). In this condition the pressure in the abdomen is increased and the neural drive to the motor neuron pool is already increased. Thus, if changes in the neural drive explain the findings of the respiratory study, then the transversus abdominis should be active earlier in the valsalva condition. However, if pre-existing abdominal pressurization provides the explanation then activation of the transversus

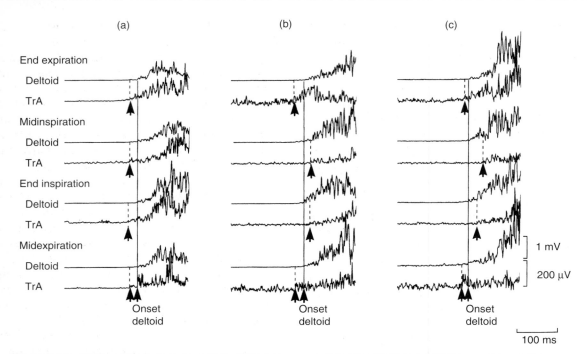

**Figure 4.12** Mean electromyographic activity of the transversus abdominis (TrA) and deltoid averaged over five repetitions for rapid shoulder flexion performed during four different phases of the respiratory cycle (end-expiration, mid-inspiration, end-inspiration, mid-expiration) with (A) relaxed breathing, (B) breathing against an inspiratory load, and (C) with forced expiration. For averaging, trials were aligned to the onset of deltoid activity, which is denoted by the solid line. The onset of TrA in each condition is marked by an arrow and a dashed line. It can be seen that the respiratory phase has no influence on the timing of feedforward contraction of the TrA with quiet respiration, but is affected by phase in the other two conditions, which resulted in increased abdominal activity during the expiratory phase. (Reproduced with permission from Hodges et al,[145] p. 757.)

abdominis should be delayed. We found that the activity of the transversus abdominis was in fact delayed, thus supporting the proposal that transversus abdominis activation is dependent on the pre-existing pressurization of the abdominal cavity.

## Summary

From all the studies described above it is becoming apparent that the transversus abdominis does contribute to spinal stability. Yet it appears to contribute to the control of non-direction-specific generation of spinal stiffness and inter-segmental control of the lumbar spine rather than the control of direction-specific forces. Perhaps most interestingly, the transversus abdominis appears to be controlled independently of the other trunk muscles. Studies are continuing in order to investigate further the control of the transversus abdominis by the CNS. How the

transversus abdominis may contribute to spinal control is the topic of the remainder of this chapter.

## CONTRIBUTION OF THE TRANSVERSUS ABDOMINIS TO SPINAL STABILITY: POSSIBLE MECHANISMS

Although the contribution of the transversus abdominis (via its role in the production of fascial tension and increased IAP) to the production of a trunk extensor moment is questionable (see Ch. 3), this muscle may be involved in the control of spinal stiffness and the inter-segmental relationship. Any contribution that the transversus abdominis makes to the control of spinal stability must involve either its contribution to the generation of pressure in the abdominal cavity or tension in the thoraco-lumbar fascia. Below we discuss each of the hypothesized mechanisms through which the transversus abdominis can influence spinal stiffness through its contribution to pressure and fascial tension.

## Conversion of the abdomen and spine to a rigid cylinder

Development of a pressurized visceral cavity through increasing IAP maintains the hoop-like geometry of the abdominal muscles (particularly the transversus abdominis).[91,116] This combined action of transversus abdominis contraction and IAP converts the abdomen and spine into a rigid cylinder. The mechanical properties of a cylinder result in a stiffer structure than the multi-segmented column of the ligamentous spine.[222,224,249] In addition, the pressurized hoop-like geometry of abdominal muscles increases the potential for lateral tension of the transversus abdominis to support the spine, in a similar manner to guy wires supporting the mast of a sailing ship.[222] Finally, several authors consider that the IAP may contribute to a posterior force, which increases the tension of the thoracolumbar fascia.[118,223]

In order to evaluate these hypotheses, the biomechanical interaction between the IAP and the thoracolumbar fascia tension requires consideration. A force balance exists between the IAP and the tensile force in the circumferential abdominal wall,[130] which can be described by LaPlace's law:

$$T = PR$$

where $T$ is the tension developed in the hoop (abdominal tension), $R$ is the radius of the arc or circle, and $P$ is the pressure developed (IAP).[7] Therefore,

Transversus abdominis hoop tension =
IAP × Abdominal radius

This means that the increased IAP may be produced either by increased tension in the abdominal wall or by a reduction in the radius of the curvature of the abdominal wall, diaphragm or pelvic floor. The estimated tension calculated using the above equation is only sufficient if the container is perfectly cylindrical and the ends of the cylinder are closed.[31] Therefore, this equation can only provide an approximation of the non-uniformly cylindrical abdominal wall.[276] Furthermore, LaPlace's law relates to non-contractile hoops, and therefore the relationship is not perfect for a muscular hoop where the magnitude of muscle force varies with the velocity of contraction, the type of contraction (e.g. isometric, eccentric, concentric) and the length–tension relationship.

Despite these limitations, the equation can be used to estimate both the tension in the wall generated by the pressure and, conversely, the pressure generated by active tension in the muscle wall. The pressure is exerted equally in all directions, and wherever the abdominal contents meet a solid boundary the pressure exerts a force at the boundary[243] that contributes to the distending force and abdominal wall tension.[276] Obviously, the tension in the abdominal wall may be increased by an increase in the IAP (as long as the radius does not decrease) or an increase in the radius (as long as the pressure is not reduced). Therefore, the development of IAP enables the abdominal muscles to contract without collapsing into the viscera.[178,222] Minimal tension will be developed if the radius of the abdominal wall reduces concurrently with abdominal muscle contraction. Since the abdominal contents are relatively incompressible this would occur through displacement of the abdominal contents into the thoracic cavity as a result of a relaxed diaphragm. Clearly, co-contraction of the diaphragm and pelvic floor would be beneficial. However, contraction of the transversus abdominis against the gravitational stretch of the abdominal viscera allows some tension to be developed in the thoracolumbar fascia, irrespective of the IAP.

## Restriction of intersegmental motion

The transversus abdominis may also contribute to the control of intersegmental motion via production of lateral tension in the thoracolumbar fascia. By increasing the lateral tension in the thoracolumbar fascia, which acts on the transverse and spinous processes of the lumbar vertebrae, the transversus abdominis may limit

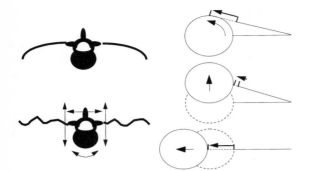

**Figure 4.13** Control of intersegmental motion via lateral tension in the thoracolumbar fascia. Motion of the vertebrae is associated with changes in the length of the fascia (right). This motion can be restrained by preventing the lengthening of the fascia. As the tensile stress in the fascia is increased, the amount of rotation and translation can be limited.

translation and rotation of the vertebrae.[148] When the joint movement occurs, the thoracolumbar fascia and transversus abdominis complex must increase in length to allow movement. Thus, when the thoracolumbar fascia is slack a certain degree of motion is allowed in all directions. As the tensile stress in the thoracolumbar fascia is increased the amount of rotation and translation is limited (Fig. 4.13). As the tensile stress increases to infinity, the available motion will reduce to zero. Through this mechanism the tension developed in the thoracolumbar fascia may limit the motion of the vertebrae in all directions. The result of this mechanism is a reduction in the size of the neutral zone, which will be optimal if the position of the transversus abdominis is stabilized. If tension is developed only in one side, then displacement may occur; however, if equal tension is developed in both sides, the motion will be restrained.

This mechanism of lumbar stability has not been previously addressed in the literature, and requires further biomechanical evaluation. However, a similar model has been suggested by McGill & Norman.[224] Their model involves the contraction of each of the abdominal muscles exerting lateral and anteroposterior forces acting as guy ropes for the spine. These authors considered that the tension developed would increase the stability and prevent buckling of the spine. Furthermore, when tension is applied to

the thoracolumbar fascia in cadavers by inflating a balloon in the abdomen, no movement occurs.[329] This supports the proposal that tensioning the thoracolumbar fascia may increase the stiffness of the spine rather than produce motion. In order for tension to be developed in the thoracolumbar fascia, the shortening of the transversus abdominis needs to be restrained. This requires containment of the abdominal contents by contraction of the diaphragm.

## Intersegmental compression

In Chapter 3 it was argued that tensioning of the obliquely oriented fibres of the thoracolumbar fascia is unlikely to contribute significantly to the production of trunk extension. However, the conversion of lateral tension to longitudinal tension via contraction of the transversus abdominis pulling laterally on the basal angle of the triangle formed by the oblique fascial fibres[116,117] is likely to produce sufficient approximating force (2% of the effective extensor torque[228]) to generate mild compression between vertebral segments. The effect of this mild compression would be control of the shear forces between segments.

Tesh and colleagues[329] proposed a further mechanism by which tension of the thoracolumbar fascia may produce a trunk extensor moment. These authors suggest that lateral tension of the fascia may produce a posteriorly directed vector acting on the interspinous ligament due to the posterolateral orientation of the fibres of the posterior layer arising from the midline structures. This was proposed to produce approximation of the spinous processes. It was estimated theoretically that the force produced by this mechanism would produce a gain of 0.22–0.64 units longitudinal force for each unit of lateral force. However, the posterior component of the force disappears as the spine is flexed.[329]

## Control of spinal stiffness in the coronal plane

The thoracolumbar fascia has also been suggested to contribute to the control of coronal plane motion via the convergence of the fibres of the middle layer of the fascia onto the transverse processes of the lumbar vertebrae.[329] It was proposed that approximation of the transverse processes would occur in a similar manner to that proposed for the production of trunk extension involving conversion of a lateral force into a longitudinal force (Fig. 4.14) (see Ch. 3). The vertical vector producing an approximation of the transverse processes has a large mechanical advantage due to the distance from the centre of rotation of the lateral flexion. Bilateral contraction of the transversus abdominis would result in a greater lateral flexion force on the convex side of the spine due to the larger angle of the fibres relative to the horizontal.[329]

The ability of this mechanism to control the spine in the coronal plane was assessed by placing cadavers in a laterally flexed position and measuring the force required to maintain this position as the tension in the fascia was

increased by inflating a balloon in the abdominal cavity.[329] The balloon was prevented from exerting pressure against the diaphragm and pelvic floor, which would simulate an increase in IAP. The maximum lateral flexion moment acting to straighten the spine as a result of this procedure was 14.5 Nm. Therefore, up to 40% of trunk stability in the coronal plane may be produced by tension of the middle layer of the thoracolumbar fascia.[329]

## IAP and the function of the spine as an arch

Several authors have considered the possibility that a posteriorly directed force on the spine resulting from the increase in IAP may stiffen the lumbar spine.[33] Aspden[21,22,23] suggested that the combined action of the posteriorly directed force and the arch-like geometry of the lumbar spine may produce a compressive effect on the convex side of the spine, resulting in increased stiffness (Fig. 4.15). This possible mechanism of spinal stability has stimulated considerable discussion in the literature. Several reports have been published questioning the capability of the spine to act in this manner on the basis of flaws in Aspden's original calculations.[4] However, it is

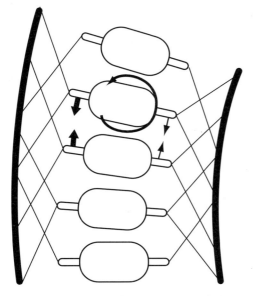

**Figure 4.14** Stabilization of the lumbar spine in the coronal plane via tension in the middle layer of the thoracolumbar fascia. The oblique orientation of the fibres of the middle layer allows lateral tension of the fascia to produce a vertical vector acting to approximate the adjacent vertebrae. When the spine is laterally flexed the magnitude of the resultant vertical vector is greater on the convex side, potentially contributing to the return of the spine to the neutral position. (Adapted from Tesh et al,[329] p. 504.)

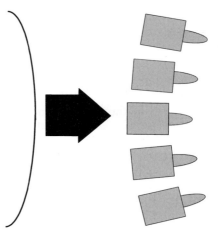

**Figure 4.15** Proposed contribution of intra-abdominal pressure to spinal stability by providing a compressive stress on the convex surface of the lumbar lordosis, which has a stiffening effect on the arch-like structure of the spine.

likely that this mechanism may make some contribution to spinal stiffness.

## Stiffness of the abdominal contents and control of intersegmental motion

When the IAP is increased the stiffness of the abdominal contents is also increased. It has been suggested that increased abdominal stiffness may assist in maintaining the alignment of the intervertebral joints by minimizing or eliminating small movements between adjacent vertebrae by a hydraulic effect.[222] How much this mechanism contributes to spinal stiffness is unknown.

## Rotatory control of intersegmental motion

A final potential contribution of contraction of transversus abdominis to the stabilization of the trunk is the potential for this muscle to produce rotation.[64] Cresswell et al[64] considered that the transversus abdominis may compensate for unequal levels of activation of the right and left obliquus externus abdominis and internus and rectus abdominis. Although the mechanism through which the transversely oriented fibres of the transversus abdominis can produce rotation is not obvious, it is possible that this muscle may contribute to the control of rotation via its attachment to the contralateral oblique muscles or via oblique fascial attachments to the linea alba. Alternatively, the transversus abdominis may contribute to rotation from a rotated position by increasing tension in the thoracolumbar fascia (see Fig. 4.13). Further investigation of the contribution of the transversus abdominis to the production of rotation is required in order to assess the viability of this proposed mechanism.

## Control of stability of the sacro-iliac joint

As outlined in Chapter 2, the mechanism of stability of the sacro-iliac joint is dependent on compression between the ilia and the sacrum (i.e. force closure) in addition to the shape of the joint surfaces (i.e. form closure).[312] Due to the

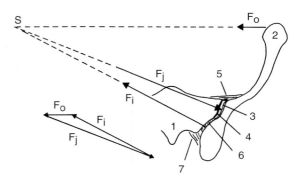

**Figure 4.16**  Cross-section of the pelvis at the level of the sacro-iliac joints. The application of force by the transversus abdominis and oblique abdominal muscles ($F_o$), in combination with stiff dorsal sacro-iliac ligaments ($F_i$), compresses the sacroiliac joints ($F_j$). Because the lever arms of the muscle and ligament force are different, the joint reaction force is much greater than the muscle force. (1) Sacrum; (2) iliac bone; (3) joint cartilage; (4) joint space; (5) ventral sacro-iliac ligament; (6) interosseous sacro-iliac ligaments; (7) dorsal sacro-iliac ligaments. (Reproduced with permission from Snijders et al,[312] p. 423.)

anterior attachment of the transversus abdominis (and the obliquus internus abdominis) to the iliac crest, this muscle is ideally placed to act on the ilia to produce compression of the sacro-iliac joints anteriorly. Due to the lever arm of the ilia, the force generated by the transversus abdominis is amplified by a factor of 4 (Fig. 4.16), thus contributing effectively to the stability mechanism of this joint.[312]

## The obliquus internus abdominis and local spinal stability

The contribution of the obliquus internus abdominis to the local stability mechanism has been relatively ignored in this section. However, some similarities between the transversus abdominis and the obliquus internus abdominis have been identified in specific experimental situations. For example, the obliquus internus abdominis is active in a feedforward manner with certain directions of movement in a limb-movement task.[148] However, a separate control of the obliquus internus abdominis has not been identified as it has for the transversus abdominis.[152] The mechanism by which the obliquus internus abdominis may contribute to stability relates to the posterior attachment of this muscle to the lower lumbar section of the thoracolumbar fascia in some people.[38] Thus, any mechanism by which the transversus abdominis contributes to stability via tensioning of the thoracolumbar fascia may be assisted by the obliquus internus abdominis at the lower lumbar levels.

## Summary

From this review it should be apparent that many possibilities exist for a contribution of contraction of the transversus abdominis to the generation of stiffness of the lumbar spine and the control of intersegmental motion. Each mechanism is consistent with the findings of direction insensitivity highlighted in the studies presented in the first section of this chapter. The amount that each mechanism contributes to spinal stability is as yet unknown. However, several research groups are currently investigating the potential of each mechanism to maintain spinal stability. Further information should be forthcoming. An important factor of many of the mechanisms is the possibility for contraction of the lumbar multifidus to contribute to tensioning of the posterior layer of the thoracolumbar fascia, since it is contained within the sheath formed by the fascia. This shared function of the transversus abdominis and lumbar multifidus has interesting implications for the optimal functioning of the spinal stability system.

# 5

# Local muscle dysfunction in low back pain

The transversus abdominis and lumbar multifidus were studied in more detail in back pain patients in an attempt to decipher the clinical evidence and to demonstrate more clearly the nature of the problem which develops in these muscles. Other researchers were also beginning to investigate the dysfunctions present in these muscles in low back pain patients.[258] The research on the local muscle system provided the foundation for new treatment methods to reverse the dysfunction in these muscles in back pain patients.

## DYSFUNCTION OF THE TRANSVERSUS ABDOMINIS

### Changes in motor control

The new knowledge of the normal function of the transversus abdominis and its contribution to spinal segmental stabilization strengthened the assumptions made from our clinical tests that transversus abdominis function was poor in patients with low back pain. The methods developed to evaluate the normal function of the transversus abdominis provided a way to evaluate closely the function of this muscle in people with low back pain. This chapter reviews these studies. The findings provide a basis for many aspects of the approach to rehabilitation of the deep, local muscle system.

### Delayed activation

Previously, in a group of people with no history of low back pain we had identified that con-

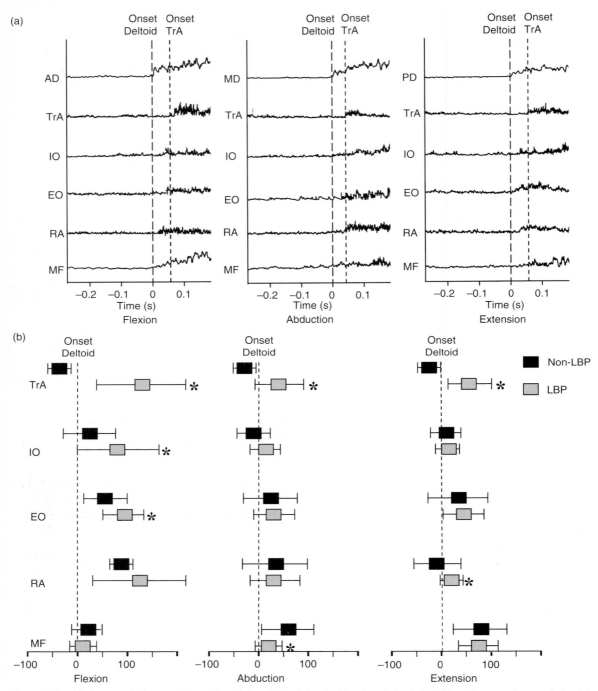

**Figure 5.1** (a) Averaged electromyographic activity of the abdominal (rectus abdominis (RA), obliquus externus abdominis (OE), obliquus internus abdominis (OI) and transversus abdominis (TrA)), superficial multifidus (MF) and deltoid (anterior (AD), middle (MD) and posterior (PD)) muscles of a representative low back pain subject with shoulder flexion, abduction and extension. (b) Mean (± SD) time of onset of electromyographic activity of each trunk muscle averaged across all low back pain (LBP) subjects ($n = 15$). The time of alignment of the data at the onset of activity of the deltoid is at zero. This figure demonstrates the delayed contraction of the TrA with shoulder movement in each direction, and delayed activation of the other trunk muscles only with specific directions of shoulder movement. (Reproduced with permission from Hodges & Richardson,[146] pp. 2645–2646.)

traction of the transversus abdominis preceded the onset of contraction of the muscle producing movement of either the arm[148] or leg.[147] The experimental model developed in these studies provided the basis to investigate the control of the spine in people with low back pain in an automatic way (i.e. free from conscious volition). We set out to identify whether any changes occurred in this anticipatory contraction in people with a history of low back pain. Subjects included in this study and those reported in the following sections were selected on the basis of clinical criteria due to the difficulty in identifying a homogeneous group on the basis of specific pathological diagnosis. Most importantly, the patients had to have had pain for at least 18 months, to have had time off work, to have sought medical or allied health intervention and to be in a period with relatively minimal or no pain at the time of testing. The procedure was identical to that outlined previously (see Ch. 4), with electromyographic (EMG) recordings made from the deep abdominal muscles with fine-wire in-dwelling electrodes. In the first study, sub-

jects performed movement of the arm into flexion, abduction and extension in response to a light. The most obvious deficit in the subjects with low back pain was the significant delay of between 50–450 ms in the onset of contraction of the transversus abdominis (Fig. 5.1). Thus, contraction of the transversus abdominis was absent from the pre-movement period, failing to prepare the spine for the perturbation resulting from limb movement. Since the task only lasted approximately 200 ms, in many trials the contraction of the transversus abdominis occurred after the movement was completed. In every trial the contraction of the transversus abdominis failed to occur prior to that of the deltoid (the muscle responsible for initiation of limb movement). This change could not be explained by the reduction in limb movement velocity, since movement was performed at the same speed by both groups.

The delay in the onset of activity of the transversus abdominis, as shown by EMG, was apparent for movement in all directions and, notably, there was also a large increase in the

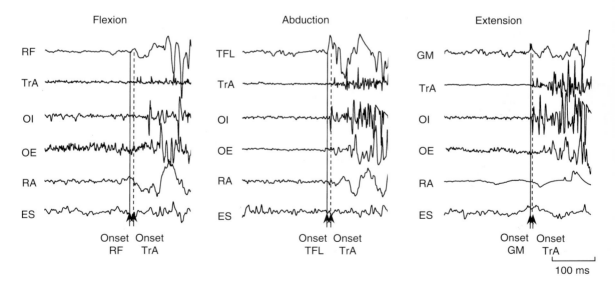

**Figure 5.2** Raw electromyographic activity of the abdominal (rectus abdominis (RA), obliquus externus abdominis (OE), obliquus internus abdominis (OI) and transversus abdominis (TrA)), superficial multifidus (MF) muscles and the prime movers of hip flexion (rectus femoris (RF)), abduction (tensor fascia latae (TFL)) and extension (gluteus maximus (GM)) with hip flexion, abduction and extension performed by a patient with low back pain. The onset of activity of the prime mover of the limb is denoted by a line and TrA is denoted by a fine dashed line. This figure demonstrates delayed onset of the TrA, occurring after that of the prime mover. (Reproduced with permission from Hodges & Richardson,[150] pp 46–56.)

variability of the response of the transversus abdominis, with large variation between subjects and between trials within a subject. The change in timing was not confined to the transversus abdominis. Delayed onset of activity was also identified for the obliquus internus abdominis, obliquus externus abdominis and rectus abdominis, although this only occurred with specific directions of limb movement.

When the same study was performed, but for movement of the leg, an identical change in anticipatory trunk muscle activity was identified by EMG.[150] Movement of the leg in all directions was associated with delayed contraction of the transversus abdominis (Fig. 5.2). Although activation of this muscle preceded the prime mover of the leg by a mean of 110 ms in people with no history of low back pain, when people with a history of low back pain performed the movement the onset of activity of the transversus abdominis followed that of the prime mover by up to several hundred milliseconds. The potential mechanism and effect of this delay will be discussed later.

## Direction-specific contraction

In patients with low back pain the onset of activity of the transversus abdominis is delayed with movement of a limb in all directions. In normal function, the transversus abdominis contracts with an identical period prior to the prime mover of the limb, with movement in all directions, suggesting that it is not responsive to changes in the direction of reactive forces acting on the spine. It was important to evaluate whether the same occurred in people with low back pain.[146] In contrast to the control group, it did not (Fig. 5.3). The contraction of the transversus abdominis was delayed by a greater period in shoulder flexion than the other movement directions. In other words, the transversus abdominis began to respond in a similar manner to the other abdominal muscles which control direction-specific forces acting on the spine. Since the transversus abdominis is unable to control direction-specific forces, the reason for this change is unclear. All other trunk muscles

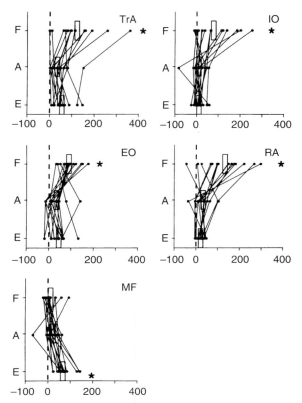

**Figure 5.3** Low back pain subject group mean (open boxes) and individual subject data (joined dots) for times of onset of electromyographic activity of each of the trunk muscles relative to the onset of deltoid with shoulder flexion (F), abduction (A) and extension (E). Time of alignment is the onset of deltoid activity at zero (denoted by the dashed line). The individual muscle is shown in the upper right corner. Note the significantly earlier onset of the transversus abdominis (TrA) with shoulder extension, which is in contrast to the control group (see Fig. 4.8) and the differences in time of onset of activity of the other trunk muscles consistent with the control group. *$p < 0.01$. IO, obliquus internus abdominis; EO, obliquus externus abdominis; MF, multifidus; RA, rectus abdominis. (Reproduced with permission from Hodges & Richardson,[146] p. 2645.)

evaluated showed identical direction-specific activation patterns as had been identified for subjects without low back pain (controls). Once again the transversus abdominis was the muscle most affected in people with low back pain. The change in control has further implications for the understanding of the mechanism of contraction of the transversus abdominis.

## Phasic contraction

An additional observation in the low back pain subjects that was not evaluated specifically in the reported data was the pattern of activity, as seen on EMG, of the trunk muscles. Observation of the raw EMG traces demonstrated an interesting finding. In contrast to the tonic postural response of the transversus abdominis in the control group, this muscle appeared to respond in distinct phasic bursts in low back pain subjects.[146] When shoulder flexion was performed the transversus abdominis responded in a single short-duration burst, along with the flexing abdominal muscles. In shoulder extension the transversus abdominis responded with two distinct bursts, once again in phase and similar to those of the flexing abdominal muscles. This change in burst pattern provides further indication of a change in control strategy employed by the central nervous system (CNS) to control activation of the transversus abdominis, and highlights the loss of tonic or isometric function of the transversus abdominis in low back pain. A similar loss of tonic function was highlighted previously in the vastus medialis oblique in a group of people with patellofemoral pain.[277,278]

## Loss of independent control

With the evidence that the motor control of the transversus abdominis is altered in people with low back pain (i.e. there is a change in direction-specific control), we then investigated the extent of these changes in more detail. This involved a similar methodology to that described previously for normal subjects, where the preparatory set of the subject was varied by providing correct, neutral or incorrect preparatory information to the subjects. As was seen in the previous study,[151] the control subjects displayed a delay in reaction time of the deltoid with decreasing preparation, which was accompanied by a delay in rectus abdominis, obliquus externus abdominis and obliquus internus abdominis reaction time, but not in that of the transversus abdominis.[152] However, the low back pain subjects responded

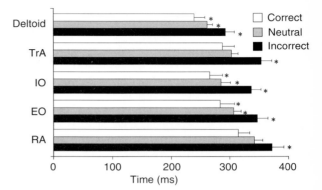

**Figure 5.4** Reaction time (mean + SEM) of the abdominal (rectus abdominis (RA), obliquus externus abdominis (OE), obliquus internus abdominis (OI) and transversus abdominis (TrA)) and deltoid muscles from a visual stimulus to the onset of electromyographic activity of each muscle with varying levels of preparation for movement (correct, neutral and incorrect) for a group of subjects ($n = 14$) with a history of low back pain. It can be seen that the reaction times of all muscles, notably including the TrA, are increased as the level of preparation is decreased, thus suggesting that the separate control of the TrA is lost in people with low back pain. $*p < 0.05$. (Adapted from Hodges & Richardson.[151])

in a different manner. The postural contraction of the rectus abdominis, obliquus externus abdominis and obliquus internus abdominis was delayed along with deltoid, as had been seen for the control subjects (Fig. 5.4). However, the onset of activity of the transversus abdominis was also delayed, along with deltoid. This suggests that, unlike the control subjects, the CNS of low back pain subjects waited until it knew what movement would be performed before it initiated contraction of the transversus abdominis. Thus, the central mechanism of transversus abdominis contraction was changed. This finding suggests that people with low back pain have changes in their postural motor control, and independent control of the transversus abdominis is lost.

## Failure to respond in natural-speed movements

In a final study we evaluated whether the threshold for activation of the transversus abdominis was modified in people with low back pain (Hodges & Richardson, unpublished results). In subjects without low back pain (controls) we had identified that anticipatory transversus abdominis

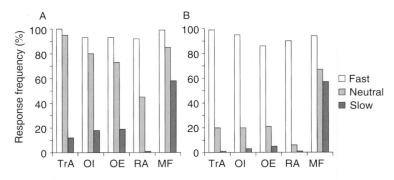

**Figure 5.5**  Frequency of trials in which a response of each of the abdominal (rectus abdominis (RA), obliquus externus abdominis (OE), obliquus internus abdominis (OI) and transversus abdominis (TrA)) and superficial multifidus (MF) muscles was present with movement of the upper limb at each of three different speeds of limb movement: fast (~ 300°/s), natural (~ 150°/s), slow (~ 30°/s), for controls (A) and patients with a history of low back pain (B). It can be seen that the frequency of response of all the abdominal muscles is reduced in the natural speed condition for the subjects with low back pain, thus suggesting that the threshold speed for trunk muscle activation is increased when people have low back pain. (Hodges & Richardson, unpublished results.)

activity occurred with movement at natural (~ 150°/s) and fast (~ 300°/s) speeds but not with movement slower than 30°/s. This suggested that the transversus abdominis responds when the reactive forces resulting from limb movement reach a certain threshold. When an identical study was undertaken on people with low back pain it was identified that a response of the transversus abdominis was only recorded when movement was performed at the fast speed (Fig. 5.5). In other words, the threshold for activation of the transversus abdominis had been increased in the low back pain patients. A similar change in threshold for activation was identified for the obliquus externus abdominis, rectus abdominis and obliquus internus abdominis. Whether this response results from changes in kinesthetic information from the joint structures, failed perception of the stability requirement or some other factors, is unknown.

## Mechanism, relevance and timing

There are three questions for which we have no definite answers and which require further investigation. First, does the delay in transversus abdominis activation occur before or after the onset of low back pain? Second, why does the timing of transversus abdominis activity and the strategy used by the CNS to control this muscle change in people with low back pain? Finally, what does the change in timing of transversus abdominis activity mean to the spine? These questions will be addressed individually.

Whether the change in transversus abdominis timing precedes the onset of low back pain or follows it is an important question. On the basis of the previous studies done by us[140] and Cresswell and colleagues,[64] which suggested a critical role of the transversus abdominis in spinal stability, it would seem possible that delayed transversus abdominis activation with arm movement may leave the spine unprotected from the reactive forces resulting from the movement. Although other types of movement have not, as yet, been evaluated, it would seem likely that the identified delay might be associated with other body movements. Failure of the spine's protective mechanism would have the potential to lead to development of microtrauma of joint structures due to uncontrolled movement. This could, hypothetically, occur as a back pain mechanism. However, it is clear that many cases of low back pain could not be attributed to such a mechanism, particularly those of traumatic origin. Obviously, longitudinal studies are required to provide evidence of a potential predisposition to back pain. The implications from such findings are particularly significant for prevention and screening.

The question of mechanism is also difficult to answer, and many studies need to be done to evaluate this question. However, there are some clues from the literature and from the specific changes we have identified. The only other studies that have successfully identified a similar delay in the onset of activity of postural muscles in association with rapid limb movement have been the evaluation of people with CNS disorders such as lesions of the frontal lobe[261] and Parkinson's disease.[203,289] The potential for dysfunction of the CNS to explain the mechanism of the delay in activation of the transversus abdominis and the other abdominal muscles seems likely from the results of the limb-movement studies. Other studies have identified a relationship between low back pain and changes in CNS parameters, including a loss of the biphasic pattern of contraction of the superficial multifidus when catching a load anteriorly.[184] In addition, other electromyographic studies have reported asymmetry[61] or abnormal levels[360] of activity of the paraspinal muscles, which has been attributed to a 'faulty neuromotor control pattern'.[84] A separate group of studies has proposed that the development of low back pain may be associated with excessive erector spinae muscle activity in response to unexpected loading of the trunk;[204,236] however, no subjects with low back pain have been assessed.

Studies of the behaviour of the CNS have identified changes in upper limb reaction time,[214,327,342] changes in the control of the position of the centre of gravity relative to the base of support[46] and changes in other parameters such as muscle tone and coordination.[162] A final group of studies has addressed the relationship between vestibular deficits and trunk muscle function, identifying an association between vestibular deficits and idiopathic scoliosis[132] and delayed onset of activity of the rectus abdominis following support surface perturbation.[9,183] A

further study linked changes in temporal parameters of the response of the gastrocnemius in a stepping task with the combined influence of vestibular deficits and low back pain.[104] Thus evidence is available to support a link between changes in control of movement by the CNS and low back pain.

Other factors may also produce deviations in the timing of onset of muscle contraction, such as a delay in postural muscle activity onset resulting from decreased limb-movement velocity.[158,207] Since the limb-movement velocity was comparable between groups, it is unlikely that this explains the present findings.[146] Another possible factor that may cause changes in the timing of muscle activity is reflex inhibition. Reflex inhibition produces a decreased activation level of the motor neuron pool,[322] and may cause delayed muscle activation as a result of the increased time taken by the motor neurons to reach the threshold for activation. Several factors resulting from musculoskeletal trauma and associated with low back pain have been linked with reflex inhibition. These include joint effusion,[78,322] pain,[318] ligament stretch[89] and capsular compression.[89] Such circumstances may influence the timing of activation of trunk muscles by lowering the excitability of the motor neuron pool. Fatigue[126] and postural variation[206] have also been suggested to influence the excitability of the motor neuron pool. However, it is unlikely that the changes in the directional specificity of the response could be explained by this mechanism. In addition, the innervation of the transversus abdominis by the T7–T12 spinal nerve makes this proposal unlikely, as the mechanism of reflex inhibition acts through a single segment of the spinal cord[322] and the structures most commonly involved in the low back pain pathology are at the L4–L5 and L5–S1 levels. The possibility of a long loop pain inhibitory mechanism[320] cannot be disregarded. Finally, the difference in magnitude of the delay in activation of the transversus abdominis identified between flexion and extension cannot be explained by this mechanism, since the influence of reflex inhibition would not be different between limb movement directions.

Another dysfunction that results in changes in the time of onset of contraction is a reduction in the conduction velocity of the motor neuron. Kleinrensink and colleagues[187] identified a delay in the reaction time of the peroneal nerve following ankle sprain, suggesting that injury to the nerve occurs in conjunction with the sprain producing the change. However, a reduced nerve conduction velocity in the peripheral nerve cannot explain the identified direction-specific differences in the transversus abdominis delay. In summary, it appears that the most likely explanation for the delay in activation of the transversus abdominis is changes in the motor control of this muscle. The implications this has for patient management are presented in Chapter 6.

The third question relates to the consequence of the delayed transversus abdominis activation for the spine. As mentioned above, theoretically the failure of transversus abdominis activation would leave the spine unprotected from the perturbation. Consequently, the spine is left unprotected, and it must be considered what structure has taken over the function of the transversus abdominis. Are other muscles trying to substitute for the function of the transversus abdominis? On the basis of muscle architecture and attachments it can be seen that no muscle, other than the lumbar multifidus, could effectively take over some of the function of the transversus abdominis. Alternatively, increased stress is placed on the passive support structures. Repeated microtrauma of joint structures has been linked to back pain.[91] No studies have been completed to address the issue of the mechanical consequences. However, with the advent of techniques for direct measurement of intervertebral motion, this type of evaluation will be possible and is essential.

## Summary

It appears that the most significant and consistent change in the anterior trunk muscles in people with low back pain is that of the transversus abdominis. Importantly, the evidence suggests that the problem is not an issue of strength or endurance but one of motor control. Surprisingly, the change in transversus abdominis control appears to occur irrespective of the specific pathology. Thus, regardless of the specific spinal structure that is involved in provoking the back pain, the changes in the transversus abdominis seem to be consistent. This question needs further investigation. The evidence for the changes in the way the muscle is controlled by the CNS is considerable and has important implications for the approach to management of the dysfunction. Obviously, limb movement is only one situation. It is likely that the change in transversus abdominis timing we have identified is only one aspect of the dysfunction in this muscle, and further investigations of other movements and types of perturbation are ongoing in our present research. In addition, further studies are required to validate further the relationship between the volitional clinical test of the transversus abdominis and transversus abdominis timing. Some attempt has been made to do this, and is outlined in Chapter 8.

## DYSFUNCTION OF THE MULTIFIDUS

There is evidence of dysfunction in the paraspinal muscles in low back pain patients, and this has been detected through measures of muscle activation, fatiguability, muscle composition and muscle size and consistency. The back extensors as a group can become dysfunctional in low back pain patients, but particular attention here will be given to the lumbar multifidus muscle.

### Muscle activation

Several general investigations of activation of the paraspinal muscles using surface EMG have discriminated low back pain patients from asymptomatic controls[51,114] by demonstrating differing patterns of activation between the groups with various tasks.[256,314] Sihvonen et al[307] studied the lumbar multifidus muscle more specifically and used EMG with surface and fine-wire electrodes to examine activation at the

L4 and L5 vertebral levels in 87 low back pain patients and 25 asymptomatic subjects during forward flexion and the return to the upright position. In addition to EMG, Sihvonen et al[307] further examined low back pain patients using plain and mobility radiographs to measure the mobility between lumbar vertebrae during trunk flexion. The activity levels in the segmental multifidus were different in the two groups. General EMG results of the raw intramuscular activity in low back pain subjects showed that during lumbar extension there was decreased activity in both segments studied when compared with controls. In the 28 of 87 patients with segmental instability, defined as a greater than 4 mm sliding between lumbar vertebrae during flexion on full-sized radiographs, the EMG results were different at different segments. There was less activity at the unstable level during concentric back activity, suggesting decreased muscular protection at the hyper-mobile level, the opposite of what is logically required.

## Fatiguability

Fatiguability infers potentially inadequate muscular support over extended periods of time. There is evidence that fatigue of paraspinal muscles is more prevalent in low back pain patients than in control subjects. Fatigue can be defined in mechanical terms as the point at which a contraction can no longer be maintained at a certain level (isometric fatigue) or when repetitive work can no longer be sustained at a certain output (dynamic fatigue).[13] Fatigue studies which have been performed on spinal muscles can be divided into mechanical studies and EMG studies.

Differences between low back pain patients and asymptomatic controls have been detected using a mechanical method of testing the isometric endurance of the trunk extensors as a group.[171,254] While no differences were detected in the trunk extensor strength between low back pain patients and controls, low back pain patients were shown to have significantly less endurance than control subjects, indicating

greater fatiguability. Such studies have a disadvantage in that they do not permit specific investigations of particular muscles within the back extensor group. The use of power spectral analysis of muscle activity as measured using EMG with multiple electrode placements has allowed assessment of individual paraspinal muscles.

In studies including the specific examination of the lumbar multifidus in low back pain patients and control subjects, differences between the fatigue rates of this muscle have been detected using power spectral analysis of electromyographic activity. Biedermann et al[34] examined the multifidus and ilicostalis lumborum in patients with chronic low back pain and demonstrated that it was the multifidus that demonstrated the greater fatigue rates in the low back pain patients compared to normal control subjects. Roy et al[290] also compared subjects with a history of chronic low back pain with asymptomatic control subjects, and again showed that the multifidus muscles of the patients demonstrated significantly higher fatigue rates than did the controls. They extended their studies and investigated high-performance athletes (male rowers). The fatigue rates correctly identified all control subjects and 93% of the subjects with low back pain.[291] As an aside from a rehabilitation perspective, it is pertinent to note that in these elite and highly trained athletes, local muscle dysfunction of the multifidus was present despite rigorous general training regimes. This supports the use of a different exercise approach to address this dysfunction in the multifidus.

## Composition

Studies based on examination of changes in type I and type II muscle fibres in low back pain patients have been conducted in order to provide insight into paraspinal muscle dysfunction. The two main parameters of multifidus muscle composition which have been examined in low back pain patients are changes in muscle fibre size and muscle fibre internal structure.

Several biopsy studies of the lumbar multi-fidus muscle have been conducted on low back pain patients undergoing lumbar surgery. Selective atrophy of type II muscle fibres has been shown,[94,98,172,239,274,365] but the significance of this atrophy to low back pain is unclear as it has also been reported in cadaveric specimens who in life had no history of lumbar disorders.[239,274] Changes in the internal structure of type I fibres of the multifidus muscle have been demonstrated in low back pain patients, although it appears that the size of these fibres remains generally unaffected.[24,98,179,239,274,365] The fibres have been described as core-targetoid and moth-eaten in appearance, and these internal structural changes are considered abnormal for healthy muscle.[239] Changes in the internal structure of type I fibres occur quickly. They have been demonstrated in biopsy specimens of subjects with a symptom duration of only 3 weeks (range 3 weeks to 1 year).[98]

The long-term sequelae of type II muscle fibre atrophy and type I internal structural changes of the multifidus have been determined in a recent study of low back pain surgery patients.[274] Muscle biopsy specimens were obtained from patients at operation for lumbar disc herniation and after a postoperative follow-up period of 5 years. Patients from the study were divided into two groups (positive or negative outcome) on the basis of their functional handicap at the 5-year follow-up. Biopsy specimens collected at operation from all subjects showed evidence of type II muscle fibre atrophy and type I fibre internal structural changes. At follow-up, results showed that no significant changes in atrophy were found in either patient group. In contrast, changes in the internal structure of type I muscle fibres showed a dramatically different result. Moth-eaten and core-targetoid fibres were seen in the initial multifidus biopsy samples of all patients. In the positive-outcome group, the presence of both these internal structure abnormalities decreased. In contrast, the negative-outcome group showed a marked increase in the frequency of these abnormalities, the increase being the greatest in moth-eaten fibres (the percentage of moth-eaten fibres increased from 2.7% to 16.7%).

The results of this study indicated for the first time that pathological structural changes in the multifidus muscle found at long-term follow-up correlated well with the long-term clinical outcome. Functional recovery after disc surgery was associated with curtailment of structural abnormalities in the multifidus muscle, especially in the type I muscle fibres. These findings highlight the potential clinical importance of dysfunction in this muscle. It seems that the pathological changes seen originally at initial biopsy could be reversed by adequate surgical and physical therapy management.

## Size and consistency

Dysfunction of the lumbar muscles in low back pain patients has also been demonstrated using imaging modalities that allow assessment of muscle size or cross-sectional area and muscle consistency. Atrophy in terms of decreased size of the paraspinal muscles has been demonstrated using imaging techniques, including computed tomography (CT) scanning, magnetic resonance imaging (MRI) and ultrasound imaging. In addition, muscle density can also be assessed with CT scanning and MRI. Decreased muscle density, which can be a sign of muscle atrophy, is caused by fatty infiltration (increased fat/muscle fibre ratio) or actual fatty replacement of fibres.[201,240] The majority of imaging studies on low back pain patients have measured these aspects for both the multifidus and the lumbar erector spinae muscles together as a lumbar paraspinal group. A few studies have investigated the multifidus in isolation from the other lumbar muscles.

### The paraspinal muscles

Several studies have provided evidence of paraspinal muscle atrophy in patients with chronic low back pain or in patients postoperatively.[6,58,159,240,267,328] In most instances this has been ascribed primarily to disuse and deconditioning.[58,159,240,267,328] Two studies have examined the paraspinal muscles of low back pain patients in more detail and have shown differences between sides and vertebral levels.[6,201]

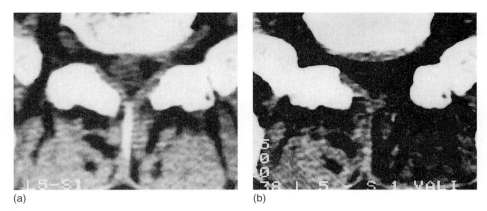

(a)                                    (b)

**Figure 5.6**   Computed tomography scans taken from the L5 to S1 level: (a) before surgery, when disc protrusion facet arthrosis and lateral stenosis at this level was noted; (b) after left hemilaminectomy was performed, showing multifidus muscle atrophy at the corresponding vertebral level (L5–S1). (Reproduced with permission from Sihvonen et al,[306] p. 578.)

In an examination of postoperative patients, Laasonen[201] showed that, when atrophy was partial, it always included atrophy of the medial portion of the multifidus. In unilateral cases, paraspinal muscles were shown to be 10–30% smaller on the affected side than on the unaffected side. Fatty degeneration of the paraspinal muscles was also evident. A positive relationship between the fat content of the paraspinal muscles at the lumbosacral junction and results of a disability index was demonstrated in chronic low back pain and lumbar postoperative patients.[6] This relationship between fat content and disability was not demonstrated at other vertebral levels, thus highlighting the fact that investigation of muscle atrophy in low back pain patients must be directed to several vertebral levels if the relevant changes are to be discovered.

### The multifidus muscle

Two groups have investigated the effects of low back pain on the multifidus muscle size specifically, using imaging modalities. One studied postoperative patients,[306] and the other acute and subacute low back pain patients.[136,139]

The direct effects of lumbar surgery (iatrogenic trauma) on the lumbar multifidus muscle was examined by Sihvonen et al.[306] They demonstrated that, in some cases, lumbar surgery for spinal stenosis and/or disc herniation could lead to severe changes in the multifidus muscle (Fig. 5.6). Two groups of subjects were studied: those with a poor outcome and those with a good outcome from surgery. It was found that patients could have similar outcomes in surgical terms via successful nerve decompression and absence of stenotic regrowth. Nevertheless, they could have different functional recoveries. A variable related to poor outcomes was multifidus muscle atrophy, which was more prevalent in patients with the poorer postoperative outcomes.

We have investigated the lumbar multifidus in patients with acute low back pain using real-time ultrasound imaging. In the first study, the cross-sectional area of the multifidus was measured in 26 patients with first-episode acute unilateral low back pain of a mean duration of approximately 2 weeks, and 51 normal subjects. In low back pain patients the muscle on both sides was measured at all vertebral levels from the second lumbar to the first sacral vertebra.[139] In the 51 normals the cross-sectional area was measured at L4, and in 10 subjects measurements were made from L2–L5. Marked side-to-side asymmetry of the cross-sectional area of the multifidus was found in the low back pain patients but not in the normal, non-back-pain subjects (Fig. 5.7). The smaller muscle was found

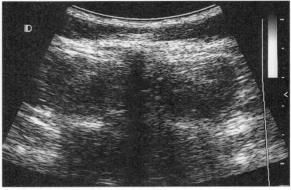

(a)

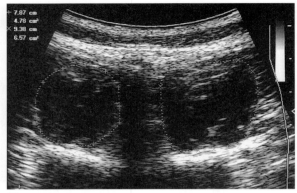

(d)

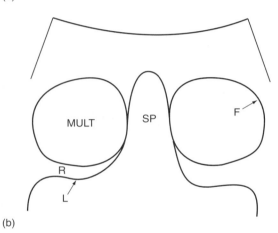

(b)

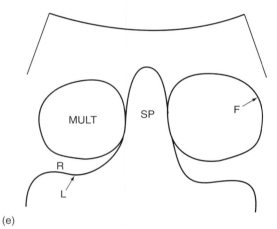

(e)

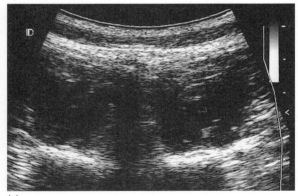

(c)

**Figure 5.7** (a) Sonographic appearance of the multifidus (axial image) at the level of the fifth vertebra in a normal subject. (b) The multifidus muscle (MULT) is bordered by the vertebral lamina/zygapophyseal joint (L) inferiorly, the spinous process (SP) medially, fascia, fat and skin superiorly, and the fascia between the multifidus and the lumbar longissimus and iliocostalis (F) laterally. The brightness seen at the interior border of the multifidus is reflection (R) of sound waves from the vertebral lamina and zygapophyseal joints. Acoustic shadowing is seen inferior to this landmark, as the ultrasound waves are unable to penetrate the bone. (c) Sonographic appearance of the multifidus (axial image) at the level of the fifth vertebra in a patient with unilateral left-sided low back pain. (d) In this image the borders of the multifidus have been traced to demonstrate the asymmetry. The multifidus on the left (symptomatic) side is 4.78 cm$^2$, while the larger multifidus on the right side is 6.57 cm$^2$. This represents a decrease on the left side of 27%. (e) Note the decreased size of the left multifidus in comparison with the right side. Labels are as in (b).

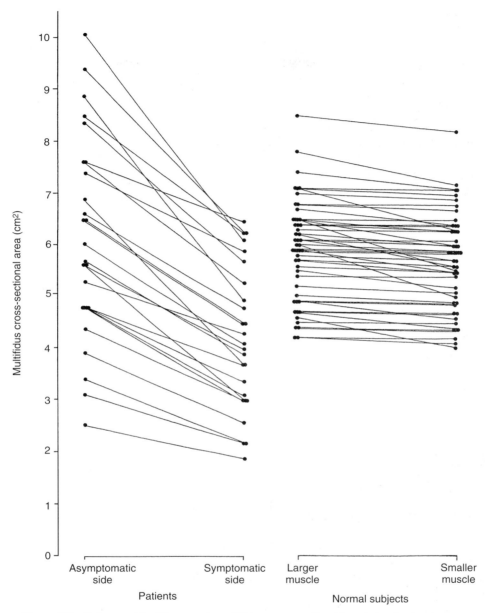

**Figure 5.8**    Between-side differences in multifidus cross-sectional area in low back pain patients ($n = 26$) who showed greater asymmetry than the normal subjects ($n = 51$). The degree of asymmetry was significantly different between the two groups ($p < 0.001$). (Reproduced with permission from Hides et al,[139] p. 169.)

at the symptomatic segment, was on the side ipsilateral to symptoms, and was confined predominantly to that one vertebral level. The magnitude of the between-side difference was $31 \pm 8\%$. In normal subjects this was $3 \pm 4\%$. This difference in asymmetry is illustrated for patients at the level of symptoms and at L4 for all the normal subjects in Figure 5.8. Such a comparison between the two groups is considered valid since the degree of asymmetry in normal subjects was similar at all vertebral levels. The changes occurred quickly. One subject was measured within 24 h of injury and displayed the asymmetry. Therefore a likely explanation for the mechanism is inhibition of the segmental multifidus.

Following on from the findings from the initial study, a randomized clinical trial was conducted. The aim of this research was to monitor if the multifidus muscle recovered spontaneously over time and to evaluate any effect of specific rehabilitation of this segmental dysfunction. Thirty-nine subjects with acute first-episode unilateral low back pain demonstrating unilateral segmental inhibition of the multifidus muscle participated in this clinical trial.[136] Patients were randomly allocated to a control (non-active treatment) or treatment group. Outcome measures for both groups included weekly assessments of pain, disability, range of motion and measurement of multifidus cross-sectional area over the 4-week intervention period. Patients were reassessed at 10 weeks and 35 subjects were interviewed at 1 year to establish long-term low back pain recurrence rates. Three-year follow-up data are currently being evaluated.

The decrease in multifidus size was localized to specific vertebral levels (Fig. 5.9). Subjects in the treatment group performed specific localized multifidus exercises (see Ch. 9) aimed at restoring the stabilization function of this muscle. Low back pain subsided in virtually all subjects, regardless of group (Fig. 5.10a, b), and there were no differences in disability scores (Fig. 5.10c) between the two groups at 4 weeks. The measures most commonly used in low back pain outcome trials demonstrated a return to normal function in 4 weeks, reflecting the well-known natural recovery of an acute episode of low back pain.

In the back pain group who underwent standard medical management (control group) the reduced size of the multifidus in the symptomatic side notably remained almost unchanged over the 4-week period of the trial (Fig. 5.11). In these control subjects, multifidus muscle recovery was not spontaneous with the

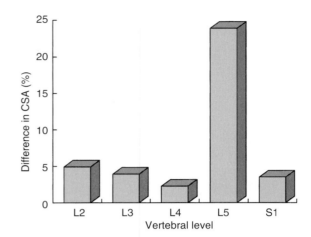

**Figure 5.9** Ultrasound imaging results showing the between-side percentage difference in multifidus cross-sectional area (CSA) for vertebral levels L2–S1 in 34 patients who demonstrated multifidus asymmetry at the L5 vertebral level. Note the greatest difference in cross-sectional area between sides at the affected vertebral level (L5) with minimal asymmetry between sides demonstrated at the other lumbar vertebral levels. (Reproduced with permission from Hides et al,[136] p. 2767.)

relief of pain. In contrast, the exercise intervention resulted in restoration of the multifidus cross-sectional area within the 4-week treatment period. Therefore, despite relief of pain and general muscle use in returning to normal activity levels, patients in the control group still displayed decreased multifidus muscle size at 4 weeks which persisted to the 10-week follow-up. Long-term results showed that only 30% of subjects from the intervention group suffered recurrences of low back pain compared with 80% of subjects from the control group.[133,137] It could be suggested that the persistence of the segmental multifidus muscle inhibition, still evident in the control group at the 10-week follow-up, exposed the injured segment to decreased muscle support and a predisposition to further injury.

This study highlights the importance of identifying and measuring the specific dysfunctions in the muscle system which are directly associated with the pain or injury. Possession of this knowledge directed very specific treatment to the dysfunctional muscle and provided a direct measure of the impair-

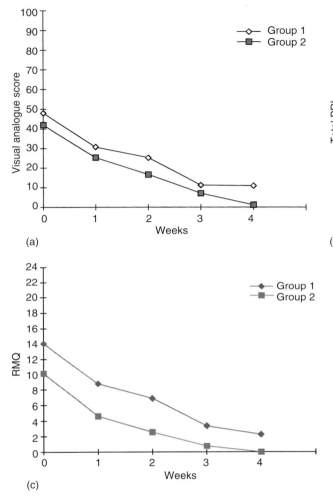

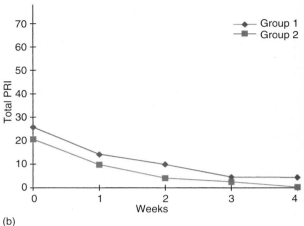

**Figure 5.10**   Pain and disability scores obtained for patients in group 1 (control group) and group 2 (specific exercise group) for the baseline measurement (week 0) and at weeks 1–4 of the study. (a) There was no significant difference at any time between pain scores obtained using visual analogue scales for the two groups. (b) There was no significant difference between pain scores on the total pain rating index (PRI) of the McGill Pain Questionnaire. (c) There was no sigificant difference in disability scores (RMQ) obtained on the Rowland Morris Disability Index. (Reproduced with permission from Hides et al,[136] p. 2765.)

ment on which to evaluate the effectiveness of the rehabilitation approach. The other commonly used outcome assessments (pain, range of motion and disability assessments) do not seem to relate to the recurrence rate of symptoms in the first year following the initial injury.

The results of this study also build on the understanding of the possible causes of the decreased multifidus size in acute low back pain patients. The possibilities include reflex inhibition, pain inhibition and disuse atrophy (see Ch. 6). The rapidity of onset and localized distribution of the decrease in muscle size suggest that disuse atrophy was not the cause. The most likely mechanism is reflex inhibition, as in our study the indirect effects of inhibition (decreased muscle size) were seen even after resolution of pain in the control group subjects.[136] Similar findings have been documented in muscles of peripheral joints, such as the knee,[164,322,324] where persistence of reflex inhibition was demonstrated well beyond resolution of painful and disabling symptoms.[198,296,322] Examination of the possible mechanism for the selective inhibition of the multifidus at the affected level is intriguing. It is the sensory innervation of the injured joint or structure which is the crucial element in reflex inhibition. Based on the sensory innervation of the knee, almost any muscle of the lower limb could potentially be

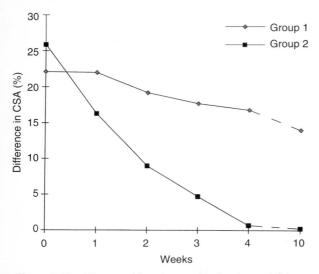

**Figure 5.11** Ultrasound imaging results showing multifidus muscle recovery for patients in group 1 (control group) and group 2 (exercise group) for the baseline measure (week 0), weeks 1–4 of the study and the 10-week follow-up examination. Muscle size is presented as the difference between sides (expressed as a percentage) in cross-sectional area (CSA) at the most affected vertebral level. (Reproduced with permission from Hides et al,[136] p. 2767.)

affected by reflex inhibition after knee injury.[182] However, it has been suggested that input from the joint is processed and modulated in the spinal cord to produce an effect in specific muscles which act on the joint in question. In the case of the knee this is the quadriceps. A similar effect appears to occur in acute low back pain.

The parts of the multifidus crossing the affected segmental level seem to be the specific parts of the muscle which are affected by reflex inhibition. Further research to gain an understanding of the possible mechanisms behind this finding of decreased multifidus cross-sectional area at the segmental level of symptoms is important to further guide appropriate rehabilitation of the segmental multifidus.

## Summary

There is a significant body of evidence that illustrates that the lumbar multifidus muscle is adversely affected in low back pain patients and dysfunction occurs with the first episode of back pain. As the multifidus muscle provides local segmental stability of the lumbar spine in normal function, dysfunction of the multifidus could be assumed to have substantial adverse effects in low back pain patients. Evidence of long-term sequelae has already been provided in post-surgery patients. Dysfunction of the multifidus has been demonstrated in low back pain patients in the areas of multifidus activation, fatiguability, muscle composition and muscle size and consistency. Information pertaining to the specific nature of dysfunction of the multifidus muscle in low back pain patients has provided a basis for the development of effective rehabilitation programmes.

# Applying science to practice

Successful treatments usually provide the direction for scientific investigations. Equally, new principles of treatment can also evolve from a research process. Careful search and enquiry into previous ideas of the pathogenesis of low back pain and its treatment and, most importantly, critical evaluation of the presentation of impairments in patients with low back pain have been used to develop the new treatment approach. This approach will always be under constant review with modifications undertaken in line with new basis science and clinical research findings.

# 6

# General considerations in motor control and joint stabilization: the basis of assessment and exercise techniques

In Section 2 we presented some of the physiological and biomechanical research which has indicated that it is the stabilizing function of muscles necessary for spinal segmental control that is a relevant and primary problem linked to low back pain. For this information to be useful, it has to be applied to clinical practice. To be efficacious, exercise methods must be able to address the normal functional role of muscle and the physiological dysfunction associated with the pain state. There are evidence-based exercise methods for increasing the strength or endurance capacity of a muscle. However, exercise that directly addresses problems in the stability function of muscles is a far more complex issue.

Joint stabilization involves an intricate inter-relationship and precise control between several muscles acting on the joint to protect it during functional movement. Relatively little is known about how individual muscles contribute to joint stabilization. Kornecki[195] acknowledges that the stability function of muscles has been neglected in general scientific research concerned with human movement. This omission has been seen in research into energy systems as well as that considering the contribution of individual groups of muscles to the production of a movement task. Therefore, at the present time, principles and methods to re-educate a muscle in its stabilization function have not been as rigorously studied, and the principles that should be followed are not universally agreed upon.

Even though research in the area of principles of therapeutic exercise for joint stabilization is sparse, an understanding of what is already known about muscle control and joint stabilization from other regions of the body will assist in the gradual development of the most effective and efficient testing and training techniques to improve spinal segmental joint stabilization. This chapter focuses on the muscle control involved in normal joint stabilization, as well as the changes in muscle control that occur with joint pathology, injury or improper use of the muscle. In investigating the links between motor control and active joint stabilization, the clinical relevance of each aspect of motor function linked to stability is addressed.

## MUSCLES THAT MOVE MORE THAN ONE JOINT

Skeletal muscles can be categorized as mono-articular, biarticular or multijoint muscles. Their capacity to provide stabilization for individual joints differs in each category and this has implications for exercise design for rehabilitation.

Muscles crossing one joint only and classified as monoarticular muscles have close associations with joint stabilization. This is reflected in their anatomical attachments. They may lie within a large synergistic group of muscles, but their individual contraction affects only one joint or, in the case of the spine, one region. Examples of such muscles are the vasti at the knee and the gluteus medius at the hip. The anatomical arrangement of these muscles enhances their joint stabilization role. They are often pennate, with extensive fascial attachments, a design linked to controlling large joint forces rather than controlling large ranges of movement.[355] They are responsible primarily for one action of the joint, i.e. they control one specific joint movement. In most cases their action is ideal for antigravity function; they control the movement of the joint when it comes under the influence of gravity.

In contrast, muscles capable of moving and to some degree supporting several joints at the same time have functional qualities that render them less able to provide individual joint sup-

port. Such multijoint muscles of the global system usually form part of a synergistic functional group of muscles. They are capable of influencing more than one joint or, in the case of the spine, more than one region (e.g. the thoracic and lumbar spines) simultaneously. Examples of such muscles in the appendicular skeleton include the rectus femoris acting on the hip and knee, the tensor fasciae latae executing various movements of the hip as well as the knee, and the latissimus dorsi, which is involved in both scapular and shoulder movements. In the spine, muscles include the thoracic erector spinae, the tendons of which in the main span the lumbar area to insert into the ilium and sacrum and, anteriorly, the rectus abdominis. Both groups influence thoracic and lumbar movement simultaneously.

In general, multijoint muscles are anatomically designed for complex movement function involving several areas of the body.[340] Their long, usually fusiform, shape together with their location, which is often remote from the joints they act upon, make them less suitable for stabilization and control of individual joints and more suitable for controlling large ranges of movement.[355] Their action is movement dependent, and is considered to be linked to the skill component of the task.[340] Multijoint muscles provide an efficient muscle system for completing a functional task. They are readily activated in movement patterns,[245] most particularly it seems in ballistic, skilled movement.[279] Clinically, multijoint muscles are more likely to become overactive and tight.[163]

In studying the stability role of muscles, the interrelationship between muscles controlling one joint and the often used and efficient multijoint muscles needs to be considered. These two functionally different types of muscle usually lie within the same functional muscle group. For stability and joint support, muscles that control one joint or region only should be closely monitored to ensure they are functioning well. The often overactive multijoint muscles should be observed to ensure they are not substituting for the work of those muscles that are more ideal for providing joint support. (See Box 6.1.)

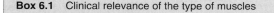

## MUSCLES SPECIALIZED FOR A JOINT STABILIZATION ROLE

There is evidence that some muscles, rather than contributing to movement of a joint system, are designed for joint stabilization. These muscles are those described by Bergmark[33] as local muscles. A good example is the vastus medialis obliquus of the knee. It was considered an extensor of the knee, but the anatomical and electromyographic studies performed by Lieb & Perry[210,211] confirmed its role, not as a knee extensor, but as a muscle designed to control and support the patella during knee movement. With reference to the trunk, McGill[219] provided evidence that the deep fibres of the lumbar multifidus undergo only minimal changes in length throughout the range of motion. This is due to their close proximity to the centre of rotation of the lumbar joints and suggests that this specific component of the back muscles contributes minimally to the production of motion. In addition, due to the transverse orientation of the muscle fibres of the transversus abdominis, biomechanically it cannot contribute to extension, flexion or lateral flexion of the spine, although it has been argued by some to contribute to some extent to trunk rotation.[64] Thus the transversus abdominis and lumbar multifidus, like the vastus medialis obliquus of the knee, have primary roles that do not include the production of motion.

Thus it can be argued that local stability muscles do not usually take part in the movement of the underlying joint, but rather directly support it while movement is occurring. These local stability muscles are usually deep and located close to the joint. They often have extensive attachments to the passive joint struc-

tures, including the joint capsule. While such muscles may only be able to generate small forces, their short length compared to the larger torque-producing muscles make them ideal for increasing joint stiffness, and hence for providing extrinsic mechanical stability to the joint they span. Examples of muscles involved in stabilization of the peripheral joints include: the muscles of the rotator cuff in the shoulder, which act like dynamic ligaments to control humeral head position;[70] the vastus medialis obliquus at the knee, which controls patellar position;[210,211] and the posterior portion of gluteus medius in the hip, which controls the femoral head in the acetabulum.[113] In the spine, muscles such as the deep longus capitus, longus colli, semispinalis cervicus and segmental multifidus are well designed to provide stability to the cervical spinal segments,[57,241,344,356] while the lumbar multifidus and transversus abdominis are capable of controlling joint stiffness in the lumbar region (see Chs 3 and 4).

Functionally, the nervous system could be expected continuously to modulate activity in these muscles in order to control joint position, irrespective of the direction of movement. In this way such muscles could provide concentrated joint support while, independently, the larger torque-producing muscles control the acceleration and braking movements of the joint.

Initial evidence that this is the case has come from our research into fast ballistic repetitive movements of the knee.[279] During rapid flexion and extension of the knee in a simulated minimal weight environment, the multijoint muscles (rectus femoris and hamstrings) controlled the acceleration and deceleration of the lower leg during the knee movements. In contrast, the vastus medialis obliquus was activated continuously during both flexion and extension phases of movement (Fig. 6.1). This continuous non-phase-dependent activation of the vastus medialis obliquus suggests that this muscle is performing the role of stabilization of the patella and not movement production. Cresswell et al[64] also observed continuous activation of transversus abdominis during repetitive flexion–extension movements of the trunk

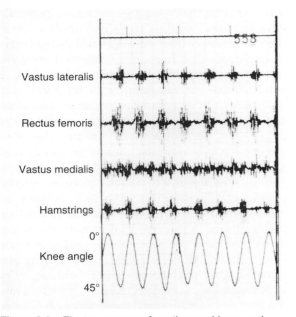

**Figure 6.1** Electromyograms from the quadriceps and hamstring muscles during rapid flexion and extension movements of the knee. Note the continuous activation of the vastus medialis obliquus during the rapidly reversing knee movement. (Reproduced with permission from Richardson & Bullock,[279] p. 56.)

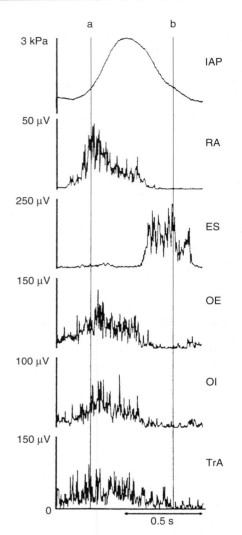

**Figure 6.2** Electromyograms from the abdominal and back extensor muscles during trunk flexion and extension. Note the continuous activation of the transversus abdominis during the reversing trunk movements. ES, erector spinae; IAP, intraabdominal pressure; OE, obliquus externus abdominis; OI, obliquus internus abdominis; RA, rectus abdominis; TrA, transversus abdominis. (Reproduced with permission from Cresswell et al,[64] p. 414.)

in the standing position (Fig. 6.2). Since the activation of the transversus abdominis was not linked to joint movement, it led these researchers to postulate a possible spinal stability role for this muscle. This stability role of the transversus abdominis is explained in more detail in Chapter 4.

This evidence supports the proposal that the deep muscles of the local system play a significant role in joint support and control during movement. This being the case, exercise training for improving joint stabilization should include methods to ensure that these muscles are capable of maintaining their activation during joint movement. (See Box 6.2.)

## LINKS BETWEEN JOINT STABILIZATION, MUSCLE STIFFNESS AND KINESTHETIC SENSE

Control of the continuous muscle recruitment for joint stability depends not only on the pre-programmed motor patterns from the cortex, but also on the state of the feedback system emanating from the kinesthetic input. The feedback system is complex and relates to the receptors within the muscle, which provide continuous information to the central nervous system (CNS) on the length and tension being

---

**Box 6.2**  Clinical relevance of muscles specialized for a joint stabilization role

- Testing and exercise procedures should include a method of recognizing if the local stability muscles are capable of supporting the joint structures.
- The procedure must include an assessment of the continuous muscle activity required for joint support for normal function.

---

generated in the muscle (for a review see McCloskey[216]). A highly sensitive and accurate information system is required to ensure the control needed to achieve joint support during functional joint movement.

Muscles behave in a similar way to a spring. They resist deformation which results from internal or external joint loading and tend to return to their original position following lengthening. 'Muscle stiffness', which is a quality reflecting the ratio of force change to length change in the muscle,[165,166] is a term used to describe the spring-like qualities of the muscle. Thus when a muscle has high stiffness, increased force is required to cause lengthening of the muscle.

Johansson et al[165,166] have undertaken much of the neurophysiological research linking muscle stiffness to joint stability. They describe muscle stiffness as having two components: intrinsic and reflex-mediated stiffness. Intrinsic stiffness refers to the viscoelastic properties in the muscle and the existing bonds between the actin and myosin. Reflex-mediated stiffness depends on the excitability of the motor neuron pool which, in turn, is dependent on the primary spindle afferents set by the degree of stretch of the muscle and the activity of the fusimotor neurons. Muscle stiffness is very closely related to the sensitivity of the proprioceptive sensory organs contained within the muscle itself.

High muscle stiffness in muscles surrounding a joint has been considered a very desirable feature to ensure good stabilization. Recently, descriptions of muscle stiffness have appeared in the biomechanical[54] and the neurophysiological literature,[165,166] with suggestions that muscle stiffness is one of the most critical variables in joint

stabilization, with low muscle stiffness generally linked to poor joint stabilization. Muscle stiffness is considered the function of muscle that is most closely related to joint protection and support, rather than the property of muscle strength or endurance. In the development of an in vivo biomechanical model of lumbar stability, Cholewicki & McGill[54] added muscle stiffness coefficients to their lumbar stability biomechanical model in order to gain more insight into muscle function associated with lumbar stabilization.

Several features of muscle stiffness can be used as the basis for understanding how muscles contribute to joint stabilization. The generation of stiffness in a muscle is linked to the activation of the tonic (postural and slow twitch) motor units (for a review see Burke & Edgerton[45]). The primary muscle afferents potently influence the small $\gamma$ motor neurons projecting to the slow twitch fibres.[167] Antigravity muscles have a large proportion of $\gamma$ (fusimotor) representation at the cortex level,[122] suggesting that fusimotor activity is a particular feature of muscles controlling the bony skeleton when under the influence of gravitational forces.

The role of muscle stiffness and feedback systems for stabilization, especially under high, unexpected loading of the joint, has always been a matter of debate. Protective reflexes have been shown to be too slow to prevent joint injury.[271] Nevertheless, Johansson et al[165,166] view the contribution of the spindle system and its fusimotor support more positively. They consider that there is a state of changeable, continuously regulated, muscle stiffness at the time of the displacement or trauma which can contribute to joint protection in unexpected loading of the joint. In the knee joint, a link has been established between receptors found in the ligaments of the joint and muscle stiffness[166] (Fig. 6.3). The sensory properties of the ligament have been shown to be related to the $\gamma$ (fusimotor) spindle system, which in turn can determine both muscle stiffness and coordination as well as movement and position sense. The $\gamma$ system appears to be the key feature of muscle stiffness. Decreased $\gamma$ support to a muscle may therefore be closely linked to poor joint stabilization.

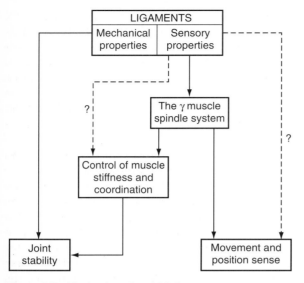

**Figure 6.3** Mechanisms by which ligaments may contribute to the regulation of joint stability and proprioception. (Reproduced with permission from Johansson et al,[166] p. 174.)

It is possible that the sensory properties of structures within the joints could be modified by the contraction of the local stability muscles. Besides providing mechanical stability to the joint, local stability muscles could also contribute to the sensory feedback mechanisms associated with the joint structures themselves, i.e. the joint capsules and ligaments. Contraction of these muscles can be associated with a tightening of these passive joint structures and thus indirectly influence their ability to detect movement. In a study involving the shoulder movement, tightening of the joint structures with active muscle contraction was found to increase the proprioceptive acuity of the joint.[35]

This knowledge of the feedback motor control mechanisms and their link to joint stabilization provides the evidence base to address muscle stiffness and proprioception when investigating muscle function associated with joint stabilization. As the tonic motor units of a muscle are linked to these factors, their contribution to the function of a muscle likewise needs to be considered. Tonic motor units are involved in tonic continuous low-load activation of the muscle.[45] This is in contrast to the strength (high load) capabilities

**Box 6.3** Clinical relevance of muscle stiffness and kinesthetic sense

Testing and exercise procedures for active joint stabilization should include:

- An emphasis on enhancing muscle stiffness and kinesthetic sensation.
- Tonic continuous low-load activation of the muscle.
- A focus on inner (shortened) range of muscle length.

of muscle function, which are linked to the phasic (fast twitch) motor units. This emphasis on low-load continuous muscle activation to enhance the ability of a muscle to stabilize joints is strengthened by recent evidence that maximum stiffness can occur at relatively low levels of maximum voluntary contraction due to the multiple factors contributing to muscle stiffness (i.e. intrinsic factors).[154] In addition, it could be argued that it is the muscle contraction in its shortened range of muscle length which is the most critical in establishing the sensitivity and optimal functional capacity of the sensory feedback system of the muscle.[284] A shortened muscle requires increased sensitivity of its spindle system, via γ or fusimotor support, to maintain the shortened length.[122] (See Box 6.3.)

## JOINT STABILIZATION THROUGH CO-CONTRACTION AND CO-ACTIVATION OF MUSCLE GROUPS

The link between co-contraction of muscle groups, usually involving the muscles on opposite sides of the joint, remains a contentious issue in relation to control of active joint stabilization. Arguments have been put forward in support of co-contraction in active joint stabilization, while others link co-contraction with rigidity, inefficiencies of muscle function and greater energy expenditure. A review of these issues is relevant when attempting to define the type of exercises that will enhance joint support.

Many consider that muscle co-contraction provides the biomechanical forces for added joint stability and joint protection,[72,218] especially in midrange, or neutral, joint positions where the ligaments and passive joint structures are more lax and hence passive restraint is minimal.[263] As a negative feature, co-contraction of muscle groups on each side of a joint has also been linked to greater energy expenditure and inefficiencies in muscle function during movement.[361] Nevertheless, the functional benefits of co-contraction need to be assessed, and these have been nominated as protection of the joint from unexpected loads, maximizing joint congruency, equalizing pressure distribution over articular surfaces, centring the joint, and stress absorption (for a review see Damiano[72]). The research done by Snyder-Mackler et al[313] adds to the case for a link between co-contraction and joint stability. Stability of the knee during gait was enhanced through electrical stimulation given in a co-contraction pattern rather than to an agonist muscle group alone.

One pertinent consideration when studying co-contraction is that all muscles of a synergistic group may not contract as a single functional entity. The larger global muscles of a group may exhibit phasic patterns during movement, while deeper muscles or parts of a muscle closer to the joint may be involved in co-contraction patterns. Supporting evidence for this pattern comes from research on the knee joint. In studies on fast repetitive knee movement, we were able to demonstrate that the phasic patterns of the hamstrings and rectus femoris were combined with co-contraction between the vastus medialis obliquus and hamstrings in one phase of the movement and the vastus medialis oblique and rectus femoris in the other phase of the movement.[279] In addition, the deep popliteus muscle in the posterior part of the knee is known to be active during weight-bearing activities of the lower limb, especially walking up hills,[27] resulting in its co-contraction with the vasti on the anterior side of the joint during such activities. This co-contraction strategy may control the rotatory stability of the knee during weight-bearing tasks. Both our clinical and basic science research is providing preliminary evidence that there is sustained co-contraction of the transversus abdominis and the deep fibres of the lumbar multifidus while the global muscles act

phasically to control trunk movement. Further research is required on movement tasks to study the extent of the co-contraction between individual muscles within and between groups for joint support during functional movement tasks. However, such research needs to include all muscle synergists, both local and global muscles, to gain true insight into the muscle patterns for joint and regional stability.

There is a large volume of research that recognizes that the neural control of stabilization includes the programming of muscles on each side of the joint to stabilize it and protect it from injury. However, the manner in which the nervous system controls co-contraction is still a matter of debate. Nielson & Kagamihara[255] suggest that co-contraction relies on a specific programme which decreases reciprocal inhibition and allows the two antagonistic muscles to increase their activity at the same time. In addition, regulation of antagonistic activity in co-contraction has been suggested to be linked to feedback loops[308] and to the cerebellum.[128]

## Co-contraction exercises

There are several issues concerning muscle co-contraction which need to be considered when planning therapeutic exercise to enhance joint control and stabilization. (See Box 6.4.).

### Inadequacy of unidirectional strength training

Unidirectional strength training of the agonist muscles can reduce co-contraction of the antagonist muscles. This was well demonstrated by Carolan & Catarelli,[50] who isometrically trained the quadriceps muscles over an 8-week period and found a significant decrease in co-contraction of the hamstrings during this time. This could be considered a serious situation, as it may compromise joint stability and predispose some population groups, such as athletes, to an increased risk of injury. Likewise, Baratta et al[25] also showed that the antagonist of a hypertrophied agonist muscle becomes markedly inhibited. Unidirectional strength training is not advisable for patients who require the control of joint stabilization through muscle co-contraction.

### Control of joint position

Co-contraction is enhanced with a focus on joint position rather than the control of force at the joint. This was confirmed by De Serres & Milner[80] in their study of muscle behaviour using the wrist as the model. Co-contraction also increased with unstable environments. Furthermore, an increase in the level of muscle co-contraction occurred with tasks that required a high degree of precision and control.[72] This occurred when there was a need for precise control of muscular tension or limb position, as well as during slow positioning tasks.

### Closed- or open-chain exercise

Muscle protection of a joint is needed in both open-chain exercise, where the distal segment moves on a fixed proximal segment, and closed-chain exercise, where the proximal segment moves on a fixed distal segment. Nevertheless, using the knee as a model, Lutz et al[215] established closed-chain exercises as a superior method to open-chain exercise to increase co-contraction of muscles surrounding a joint as well as to decrease the shear forces at the joint. This is supported by the previous findings in the knee of the potential harmful effects on stability of unidirectional strength training, which is open-chain exercise.[25]

While co-contraction is a pattern of muscle activation which appears closely linked to joint control in movement, there are some warnings. Excessively high levels of muscle co-contraction may produce harmful levels of joint compressive forces,[205,244,330] which could result in joint injury rather than providing joint protection. In addition, continuous use of inappropriately high levels of muscle co-contraction may compromise freedom of movement and cause rigidity. For this reason, co-contraction exercises may need to be directed to the local muscles specialized for a joint supporting role rather than employing and focusing on general high-load co-contraction exercises.

---

**Box 6.4**  Clinical relevance of co-contraction and co-activation of muscle groups

Testing procedures and exercise for active joint stabilization should:

- include co-contraction exercises
- avoid unidirectional (open kinetic chain) high strength training
- use slow controlled closed kinetic chain exercises
- focus on joint position rather than the control of force
- use unstable environments (e.g. a balance board)
- use slow positioning tasks which require precision and control
- include exercise in neutral joint positions
- use only low force levels for training
- not overtrain co-contraction of the large torque-producing muscle (otherwise stability may be gained while compromising freedom of movement).

---

This would be in line with the many functional situations where the local muscles will work with the agonist torque-producing muscles to provide joint protection and support through co-contraction strategies.

## FAST BALLISTIC MOVEMENT AND JOINT STABILIZATION

Logically, the muscle function that is required for fast ballistic movement is the antithesis of that required for stabilization and support of joints, but this has not been easy to demonstrate in controlled research studies. Some evidence of the relationship between fast movement and joint stabilization has come from studies involving fast movements of the knee, the ankle and the trunk.

We studied, initially in normal subjects, high-speed repeated flexion–extension movements of the knee with the load of the lower leg reduced to zero with the aid of a specially designed spring attachment[277,278] (Fig. 6.4). This exercise design was chosen because it was the antithesis to that which a physical therapist would use in stabilization training following a knee injury. As is well known, most successful rehabilitation for the quadriceps muscle involves slow, controlled, often isometric, weight-bearing exercise. The focus is on tasks for quadriceps control of knee position.[217] Fast ballistic movement, while quite

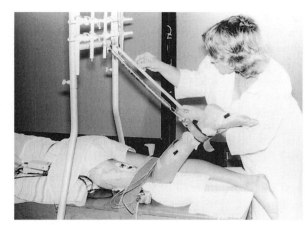

**Figure 6.4**    The exercise model used a spring attachment to reduce the load of the lower leg to zero during the high-speed ballistic task.

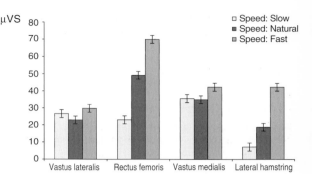

**Figure 6.5**    With ballistic exercise, note the relative increase in activity of the rectus femoris and hamstrings (multijoint muscles) when electromyographic activity was measured over three movement cycles. (Reproduced with permission from Richardson & Bullock,[279] p. 55.)

functional, is the opposite. A novel, seemingly reverse exercise design was studied via a very high-speed, non-loaded exercise that is considered to be inappropriate for re-education. This exercise design was chosen to shed some light on the possible reasons why ballistic training is not suitable and why physical therapists were intuitively prescribing the opposite for their patients. The results vindicated the non-use of high-speed exercise in early rehabilitation of the quadriceps following knee injury. We revealed that increasing the speed of knee flexion and extension, while leading to a significant increase in the levels of activity in rectus femoris and hamstrings (the multijoint muscles), had no impact with respect to increasing the relative activity levels or work in the vasti. There was no relative change in activity of the vastus medialis obliquus and vastus lateralis, the muscles which control one joint only and are responsible for stability and support in weight bearing (Fig. 6.5). In addition, these muscles displayed a continuous tonic activity to varying degrees during the phasic on/off activity of the multijoint muscles consistent with a role of control. As an aside, this finding supports Rood's[111] original classification of muscles into two joint mobilizers responsible for skilled movement, especially in non-weight-bearing, and one joint stabilizer responsible for stabilization.

Historically, Rood's classification has been used by physical therapists in exercise design.

Evidence that fast ballistic movement activates multijoint muscles preferentially to a greater extent than the one-joint muscles has also been demonstrated in studies of the lower leg and ankle joint. Increasing the speed of exercise training for the ankle plantar flexors with[252] and without weight bearing[231] led to improved function of the multijoint gastrocnemius muscle, but this was combined with a significant loss in the isometric muscle force, which could be generated by soleus, the monoarticular muscle. It is hypothesized that this change in soleus may, over time, be detrimental to the muscle support of the ankle joint, even though the skill involved in rapid plantar flexion was improving with the exercise training. Some evidence exists in the trunk of the possible effects of exercising at fast rates. Thorstensson et al[334] found an increase in rectus abdominis activity relative to the obliques in increasing speed of trunk flexion, providing some support for the generic nature of the reaction of the muscle system to ballistic training.

The muscle actions involved in fast ballistic movements tend to favour the multijoint muscles. Notably, increased activation of the multijoint, skill muscles occurs in conjunction with reduced activation of muscles which control one joint only, the muscles more likely to contribute to joint stabilization. (See Box 6.5.)

---

> **Box 6.5**    Clinical relevance of fast ballistic movement
>
> Training for active joint stabilization should:
>
> - avoid fast ballistic exercise during the early training periods
> - be implemented with caution at a late stage if required
> - involve close monitoring of the effect on local stabilizing muscles of introducing ballistic exercise.

## MUSCLE CONTROL AND JOINT PAIN AND PATHOLOGY

The muscle control necessary for joint stability is also affected by pain and joint pathology. Pain and reflex inhibition resulting from injury or pathology, in addition to a change in the sensory input to the muscles from damaged ligaments and capsules, can influence the ability of muscles to support and protect the joint. Inhibition, it will be argued, affects the tonic motor units (slow twitch fibre) in the muscles, which then become more phasic (fast twitch) in nature, compromising their supporting function. These factors need to be addressed when designing rehabilitation exercise to improve joint stabilization.

### Pain and reflex inhibition

In order to study the muscle function associated with a painful joint problem, we used the same experimental model which we used to study muscle control in fast movements of the knee in normal subjects.[277,279] The subjects were patients with patellar pain diagnosed medically as chrondromalacia patellae. With the high-speed flexion and extension, no differences from normal subjects were found in the multijoint knee flexors or extensors in their control of knee movement. However, the vasti displayed marked changes in function in these patients. Instead of the tonic (continuous) muscle activity during the phasic, on/off, activity of the multijoint muscles (See Fig. 6.1), the vastus medialis obliquus changed to work in an erratic phasic pattern similar to that seen in the multijoint muscles. This revealed that the patellar problem was linked with a failure of tonic control of the vastus medialis obliquus, but there was no change in function displayed in the multijoint muscles. In addition, the vasti increased their total activity (over three movement cycles) as the speed of the knee movement increased. This was not observed in the normal asymptomatic subjects,[279] where no change in vasti activity occurred as the speed of the movement increased (see Fig. 6.5). Therefore, in an impaired state, it can be suggested that patellar support is lost and the vasti, instead of working tonically, were acting in a more phasic manner, responding to the increases in the speed of knee movement. This change in the monoarticular knee extensors to a dysfunctional, more phasic pattern in the absence of any change in the function of the multi-joint muscles in symptomatic subjects warrants a closer examination of the effect of pain and injury on the two different muscle synergists. The findings of loss of tonic support to a more phasic pattern of muscle contraction is discussed in detail for transversus abdominis in Chapter 5.

Pain inhibition and reflex inhibition are both important phenomena that can have potent and long-lasting effects on the muscles which protect and control the joints. It is generally well recognized that musculoskeletal pain is associated with protective muscle spasm. Nevertheless, Lund et al[212] point out that pain often results in reduced levels of activity in the agonist muscle, with small increases in levels of activity in the antagonist. Reflex inhibition of a muscle has been defined as the situation that occurs when sensory stimuli impede the voluntary activation of a muscle.[250] To differentiate between pain inhibition and reflex inhibition, it has been proposed that inhibition because of pain, or fear of pain, should not be considered as reflex inhibition, which is believed to be painless.[319]

Reflex inhibition is elicited by abnormal afferent information from a damaged joint, resulting in decreased motor drive to muscle groups acting across the joint.[160] Reflex inhibition causes weakness directly and may also contribute to muscle atrophy. The joint involved is then predisposed to further damage.[322,323] This atrophy may occur rapidly.[318] Reflex inhibition is reported to hamper α motor neuron activity in the anterior horn of the spinal cord,[319] but animal studies suggest this inhibition is linked with the γ motor neuron system in inflamed joints.[127]

The sensory pathway involved in reflex inhibition involves joint afferents and articular nerves, terminating in the spinal cord. The mechanosensitivity of articular afferents is increased when joints are inflamed.[301] The pathways from joint afferents have extensive projections in the spinal cord.[60] Animal research has shown that the sensory input from the knee joint is conveyed to interneurons, motor neurons and supraspinal structures, including the cerebral cortex and the cerebellum.

The sensory pathways involved in reflex inhibition are complex. Research has been conducted on animals (mainly cats) to investigate the resultant motor reflexes.[28,86,89,105,120,157,213] Reflexes in limb muscles and reflex discharges in motor neurons can be elicited by either electrical stimulation of articular nerves or activation of receptors in the joint capsule or the joint ligaments (either directly or by pressure applied by inflation of the joint). Motor reflexes may be considered as a feedback mechanism from the joint back to the joint, since sensory information arising in the joint may influence the motor output to the muscles that move and stabilize the joint.[301]

Most research concerning patterns of muscles wasting in reflex inhibition has been conducted at the knee joint. Evidence of patterns of motor responses has been provided by the classic study of Ekholm et al,[89] which involved stimulation of joint receptors by pinching of the joint capsule. This led to inhibition of knee extensors and facilitation of knee flexors. These results have been used to explain the common finding of isolated wasting of the quadriceps with hamstring sparing in knee joint injuries. Furthermore, studies which induced joint inflammation have shown that the response to inflammation was a pronounced and prolonged increase in α motor neuron excitability in the flexor muscles.[127,362] These studies have demonstrated sensory stimuli that can exert potent effects on motor neuron excitability to a different extent in different muscle groups.

Even more specific changes have been documented. A rapid change in cross-sectional area of the lumbar multifidus at a segmental level was detected with ultrasound imaging in acute back pain patients. Hides et al[136] have argued that this change is linked to reflex inhibition (see Ch. 5). There has been an abundance of research performed on the quadriceps muscle. Studies conducted on human knee joints using experimentally induced effusions to stimulate joint receptors have shown inhibition of the vastus medialis muscle at lower magnitudes of effusion than the other vasti muscles.[182,316] Similar findings, evaluated using EMG, have been reported by Wise et al[357] in patients with patellofemoral pain syndromes. It has been reported that the rectus femoris muscle is the component of the quadriceps muscle group least affected by inhibition following injury.[318,359] This provides some explanation for the findings of Richardson & Bullock[277,278] where chondromalacia patients performed high-speed knee movement, and no changes were detected in the multijoint knee flexors or extensors. These research studies have provided evidence that reflex inhibition is likely to affect some muscles more than others. The multijoint muscles appear to be less inhibited than the monoarticular muscles.

Further evidence comes from biopsy studies. Biopsy analysis has been used in an attempt to determine the relative effects of reflex inhibition on different muscle fibre types. Susceptibility of type I muscle fibres to reflex inhibition following injury has been proposed as a possible mechanism.[123] Changes in knee muscles (antigravity muscles undergo more severe atrophy than flexors) have also been demonstrated in immobilization studies. The explanation for preferential atrophy of the vastus medialis muscle has been based on the finding that this muscle contains more type I fibres than other components of the quadriceps, making it the most vulnerable to immobilization-induced atrophy.[16] Muscles that function as antigravity muscles cross a single joint and contain a relatively large proportion of slow fibres are most vulnerable to atrophy due to immobilization.[16] This may well also be the case in reflex inhibition.

Studies conducted on the muscles of the cervical spine support the hypothesis that inhibition predominantly affects the tonic motor units (slow twitch fibre). A changing pattern of fibre type was demonstrated in patients with chronic neck pain of various pathological origins.[338,348] There was a transition in neck muscle fibre type with time in all muscles and the direction always proceeded from type I slow twitch fibres to type II fast twitch fibres. The changes did not reverse spontaneously, even with cessation of pain, and were independent of age, gender, type of pathology or the presence or not of any neurological deficit.

Clinical trials performed on human subjects highlight the devastating effects of pain and reflex inhibition. Severe muscle inhibition, demonstrated by a decrease in the maximal voluntary activation of the quadriceps of 50–70%, has been demonstrated within hours in humans using meniscectomy as a model.[322,323] Furthermore, the magnitude and duration of reflex inhibition following injury is unexpectedly high. In the study by Stokes & Young,[322,323] quadriceps inhibition became more pronounced over the first 24 h (80%) and at 3–4 days after surgery was still very severe (70–80%). Even 10–15 days postoperatively there was still 35–40% inhibition. This occurred despite the fact that patients were discharged from hospital, were experiencing minimal or no pain and were fully weight bearing. Other investigations have supported these findings with regard to the persistence of reflex inhibition.[198,296]

Ligament damage can affect sensory input to the muscles surrounding the joint and also to muscles more remote from the joint. A link has been found between damage to the cruciate ligaments in the knee and the fusimotor support to the surrounding muscles.[165,166] Injury to passive joint structures could be expected to affect both muscle stiffness and and muscle proprioception. This link between joint injury and proprioceptive deficits in the muscles needs exploration in future studies.

In addition to the muscles surrounding the injured joint, the muscles controlling more proximal joints need to be considered. Problems

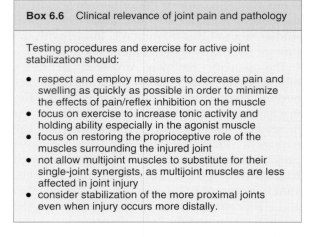

**Box 6.6**  Clinical relevance of joint pain and pathology

Testing procedures and exercise for active joint stabilization should:

- respect and employ measures to decrease pain and swelling as quickly as possible in order to minimize the effects of pain/reflex inhibition on the muscle
- focus on exercise to increase tonic activity and holding ability especially in the agonist muscle
- focus on restoring the proprioceptive role of the muscles surrounding the injured joint
- not allow multijoint muscles to substitute for their single-joint synergists, as multijoint muscles are less affected in joint injury
- consider stabilization of the more proximal joints even when injury occurs more distally.

have been found in activation of the gluteus maximus in patients with recurrent ankle ligament injuries.[44] This study emphasizes the need to assess and treat stabilization problems of more proximal joints, even when the joint injury has occurred more distally. (See Box 6.6.)

## LOSS OF MUSCLE CONTROL AND DECREASED ANTIGRAVITY FUNCTION

Loss of the stabilization function of muscles is not only associated with pain and reflex inhibition, but can also occur in circumstances of normal function. Loss of muscle control has been linked to a reduced neural input to muscles as a result of a reduction in their antigravity supporting role. Single-joint muscles are able to control joint position and are ideal for the stabilization and support of that joint. However, there are several reasons why the antigravity monoarticular muscles of a joint would be subjected to decreased neural input due to decreased use (Fig. 6.6). There are many studies which provide evidence that with decreased use or lack of use the tonic (slow twitch) fibres in the antigravity monoarticular muscle lose their characteristics and gradually change to resemble fast twitch (phasic) muscle fibres.[16,88,95,200,352,364]

While most of these studies have been performed on animal models, a study by Zetterberg et al[364] demonstrated similar changes in humans

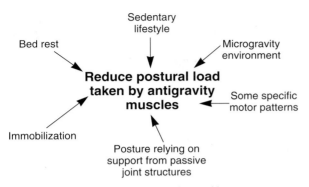

**Figure 6.6**  Reasons for decreased neural input to antigravity muscles.

<br>

**Box 6.7**  Clinical relevance of loss of muscle control and antigravity function

Testing procedures and exercise for active joint stabilization should:

- include low-load exercise (30–40% maximum voluntary contraction) to emphasize tonic continuous activity (slow twitch motor units), especially in the antigravity musculature
- change postures and movement patterns to increase the load taken by the monoarticular antigravity muscle in comparison to the multijoint synergists.

<br>

where the fibre composition of the antigravity musculature changed with reduced postural load. These researchers examined the back muscles in adolescents with scoliosis. They found an increased proportion of tonic (slow twitch) fibres on the convex side of the spine taking postural load and a decreased proportion of these fibres on the concave side of the scoliotic spine taking reduced postural load. This study provides evidence that muscles can change over time in response to a reduced postural load. A reduction in proportion of the slow twitch fibres in a muscle is likely to reduce the tonic qualities of its function (i.e. those which permit the muscle to work continuously at low levels of its maximum voluntary contraction), rather than affect the phasic (fast twitch) muscle function, which is involved in high-load and high-speed activities. (See Box 6.7.)

## CONCLUSIONS

The various aspects of motor control as they apply to the stabilization of joints have been reviewed. While stabilization training has always been a major part of the conservative management of painful musculoskeletal conditions, there have been few ways of assessing stability muscle function in the clinical setting. In developing an understanding of some of the motor control issues relating to joint stabilization, some features of clinical relevance have been highlighted which will guide clinical assessment and treatment approaches.

# Overview of the principles of clinical management of the deep muscle system for segmental stabilization

Evidence has been presented of distinct motor control problems in the deep muscles of the local system of the trunk and lumbopelvic region in patients with low back pain (see Ch. 5). In addition, there is research indicating that retraining with a specific exercise strategy can positively influence the recovery of the muscle in acute low back pain[136] and result in a better reduction in pain levels and improved functional levels in patients with chronic back pain associated with a radiological diagnosis of spondylolysis and spondylolisthesis[257].

The specific exercise strategy for segmental stabilization was developed from several sources. These included: the potential biomechanical effects of a co-contraction of the local muscles; general considerations of motor control and joint stabilization; the responses of the muscle system to training in the clinical situation; and clinical and laboratory evidence of motor control problems in the local muscles in low back pain patients. The specific exercise technique that we have developed has several special features. Some of these are similar to those found in many commonly used stabilization programmes (see Box 7.1), while others are unique, new and research based. The co-contraction exercise is best described as a specific motor skill. Persons with no history of low back pain can usually perform it quite well, but back pain patients usually experience great difficulty in attempting the skill. Such a motor skill is rehabilitated through a motor relearning process rather than through conventional exercise for increasing the strength and endurance of muscles.

**Box 7.1** The features of the specific exercise techniques

Features in common with some other stabilization programmes:
- Rehabilitation of motor control aspects of muscle function
- Neutral spine postures
- Low level continuous tonic contractions.
- Co-contraction of trunk muscles (which would include the transversus abdominis and lumbar multifidus).

Additional features of this specific exercise approach:
- Precise co-contraction of the transversus abdominis and multifidus independently of the global muscles.
- Utilization of methods of decreasing global muscle activation to allow training of the deep muscle co-contraction.
- Utilization of new facilitation strategies to achieve the deep muscle co-contraction.
- The selection of a particular treatment strategy is based directly on the assessment of the presenting impairment in the individual low back pain patient. Treatment will vary from patient to patient.
- The selection of treatments is continually being refined as their effectiveness is quantified objectively.

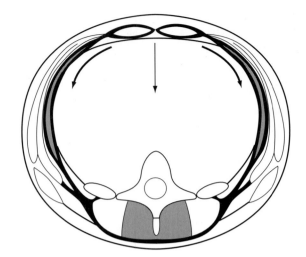

**Figure 7.1** Diagrammatic representation of the muscle contraction of 'drawing in' of the abdominal wall with an isometric contraction of the lumbar multifidus. The interrelationship and the interaction between these two muscles and the fascial system can be appreciated, and the diagram illustrates how they can work together to give spinal support.

## THE CONCEPT OF THE SPECIFIC EXERCISE STRATEGY

The concept of the exercise strategy was based historically on gaining a co-contraction of the key local muscles, the transversus abdominis and the lumbar multifidus. The aim was to effect local spinal segmental support either by the action of these muscles in increasing tension in the thoracolumbar fascia and increasing the intra-abdominal pressure (IAP), or through their direct attachment to the lumbar vertebrae. The exercise is an isometric contraction of the transversus abdominis elicited by drawing in the abdominal wall[202] combined with an isometric contraction of the segmental levels of the lumbar multifidus. Biomechanically it would be beneficial for these muscles to co-contract, and there is clinical and preliminary experimental evidence that this occurs. In the clinic it is observed that a normal cognitive contraction of the transversus abdominis is accompanied by a contraction of the lumbar multifidus and, conversely, a normal cognitive contraction of the lumbar multifidus is accompanied by a contraction of the transversus

abdominis. We propose that there is a very specific and specialized relationship between these two muscles, and it is their combined effect which is required in rehabilitation. The stabilizing effect of the co-contraction is depicted conceptually in Figure 7.1. This muscle co-contraction can be likened to activating a deep muscle corset to support the spinal segments and lumbopelvic region.

Other essential features of the exercise are the level and type of muscle co-contraction. Several factors dictate that the contraction be a low level, tonic, continuous contraction less than 30–40% of maximum voluntary contraction (MVC), with no rapid, phasic contractions (see Ch. 6). Research using electromyography (EMG) with fine-wire electrodes currently being undertaken in our laboratory has indicated that the co-contraction exercise does activate the transversus abdominis at relatively low levels in normal subjects. The exercise is isometric, with a slow and gradual development of tension to bring the muscles into their shortened range. The isometric nature of the exercise meets the functional characteristics of these muscles, as they demonstrate minimal length changes in different spinal positions and movements (see Ch. 3). The deep muscle co-contraction must be performed without substitution from larger torque-producing muscles spanning the region (e.g. the rectus abdominis, obliquus externus abdominis and thoracic portions of the erector spinae), which we have observed clinically to become overactive in low back pain patients (see Ch. 9).

Two other muscle groups are activated in synergy with the transversus abdominis and lumbar multifidus during the action of drawing in the abdominal wall. Initial data from motor control studies of trunk muscle activity in a stabilization model[141] have linked the timing of the activity of the transversus abdominis and the diaphragm. In addition, preliminary studies on the pelvic floor muscles have indicated that these muscles co-activate with the transversus abdominis (see Ch. 4). Thus, conceptually, the transversus abdominis forms the walls of a cylinder while the muscles of the pelvic floor and diaphragm form its base and lid, respectively (Fig. 7.2). This co-activation of the transversus abdominis and the muscles of the pelvic

floor and diaphragm is likely to act to maintain the IAP at a critical level, thus allowing contraction of the transversus abdominis to affect spinal support (see Ch. 4). There is some initial evidence that these four muscles act in synergy to provide a spinal support mechanism. Nevertheless, further research is required to confirm the relationship between these muscles.

It may be possible to gain some indication of ideal diaphragm activity during the specific co-contraction exercise. Historically it always appeared necessary for the patient to be able to breathe normally during the performance of the exercise strategy. New knowledge of the diaphragm's stabilization role may provide an explanation of the relevance of this normal breathing pattern. Any problem in re-establishing a normal breathing pattern with the contraction of the transversus abdominis and multifidus may indicate that the dual role of the diaphragm of contributing to trunk stabilization while controlling breathing patterns may have been interrupted in the back pain patient. More research is needed to investigate this important relationship. Nonetheless, the interaction of the muscles is used in facilitation strategies for management of the deep muscle dysfunction.

When considering overall spinal support, the local muscles can be considered as an inner corset or inner sleeve of musculofascial support. The outer sleeve comprises the global muscles and their fascial attachments. The inner sleeve is distinct from and independent of the outer sleeve, both anatomically and functionally (Fig. 7.3). Motor control studies on the action of the

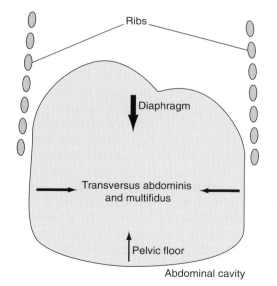

**Figure 7.2**   The functional unit of local stabilization: a stylized drawing of the transversus abdominis, diaphragm and lumbar multifidus and pelvic floor.

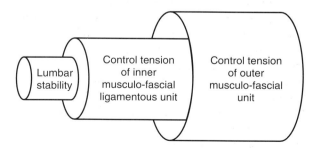

**Figure 7.3**   A conceptual model of training for stabilization of the lumbopelvic region. The inner layer is trained to provide segmental stabilization, while the outer sleeve is trained to provide a more general lumbopelvic stability function.

---

**Box 7.2**  Essential elements of the specific exercise strategy

- The focus is on the local muscles, the transversus abdominis and the segmental levels of the lumbar multifidus.
- Low load, tonic isometric contractions.
- Contraction of the pelvic floor muscles forms part of the motor skill test of drawing in the abdominal wall.
- The patient must be able to breathe normally during the abdominal drawing in action.
- Maintain specificity of deep muscle action independent of the global muscles.

---

transversus abdominis have further clarified the concept of an exercise which focuses on the co-activation of four muscles of the inner sleeve as a functional unit. The transversus abdominis acts independently of the other abdominals, thus inferring it has a separate control system. This gives a strong rationale for training the inner muscle sleeve independently of the global muscles. By its nature, the specific deep muscle co-contraction exercise could be regarded as a specific motor skill because it involves the accomplishment of a motor task with precision[52] and without the involvement of the global muscles of the outer sleeve of support. (See Box 7.2.)

# RELEARNING THE MOTOR SKILL
## Motor control problems in back pain patients

Problems in motor control of the transversus abdominis have been clearly demonstrated in terms of delayed timing of onset as well as a lack of continuous contraction during phasic activation of the main trunk torque producers (see Ch. 5). These studies have confirmed that the deficit is directly related to how this muscle controls the spine during movement. An argument for the presence of a motor control deficit in the segmental levels of lumbar multifidus muscle comes from indirect evidence at this time. This indirect evidence is based on the successful treatment of this deep muscle dysfunction,[136,257,259] where the therapeutic strategies used were consistent with those used to reverse problems

of motor control. The treatment strategy involved repeatedly practising the specific motor skill of drawing in the abdomen with a swelling of the segmental multifidus without contraction of the global muscle system. No general strength or endurance training of trunk flexors or extensors was involved in the treatment programme. The motor skill which was practised with high repetition changed the size of the inhibited levels of the multifidus in acute back pain patients quite quickly, in some patients within a week.[136] With this time frame, it can be surmised that the exercise effect was not related to muscle hypertrophy,[247] but perhaps to neurally related events in the muscle which re-established its size as well as its control of the associated lumbar segments.

## Specificity of the motor skill linked to deep stabilizing function

From the evidence that the primary problem in the deep muscles relates to their motor control and not to factors such as strength, it is proposed that the abdominal drawing in action, with its clinically observed associated lumbar multifidus activation, becomes the specialized motor skill which is linked to the stabilization capacity of these deep muscles. When evaluating people with and without low back pain performing a clinical test of transversus abdominis activation and a limb-movement task, we have shown that back pain patients with demonstrable motor control deficits in the transversus abdominis cannot successfully perform the abdominal drawing in action, whereas those without back pain who had no delay in transversus abdominis activation could readily activate the muscle.[153] Therefore, the abdominal drawing in action with its associated lumbar multifidus activation becomes the ultimate skill which needs to be learned in rehabilitation to ensure that the local muscles can perform their spinal support role. Notably, these muscles appear to be the only muscles capable of providing support at the lumbar segmental level. The other trunk muscles, which lack direct attachment to the lumbar segments, cannot substitute to perform this particular task. This reinforces the need for specific muscle assessment and training for motor control problems related to joint stabilization. The situation is completely different for most functional movement tasks where several different muscles are capable of achieving the same results. In such cases, a focus on specificity of individual muscle actions is not required for achieving a good functional outcome.

### A precise motor skill without error

Confirmation of the need for the relearning strategy to be completed very precisely, without error, has come from the motor control studies performed on chronic low back pain patients (See Ch. 5). In a dysfunctional state, the transversus abdominis changes its role from one of support, for which it is designed anatomically, biomechanically and physiologically, to one of trunk movement. Instead of continuously modulated activity, independent of the other abdominal muscles, the transversus abdominis behaves in a manner similar to the other abdominal muscles and works with trunk flexors. Therefore the exercise techniques for re-establishing its role as a deep stability muscle of the lumbar spine must, of necessity, be very precise. They must be able to change the impaired motor control where the transversus abdominis works with all abdominal wall muscles to return it to the state where it functions completely separately from the other abdominal muscles.

### Analysis of learning a precise motor skill

The principles involved in relearning a specific motor skill are very different to those for strength and endurance training. Charman[52] defines improvement in skill as being 'inversely proportional' to the amount of unnecessary muscle activity that occurs during its performance. In context, improvement in the abdominal drawing-in action by the local muscles can be rated by decreasing global muscle activity. The point is reached as the skill is perfected where no unwanted muscle activity occurs, i.e. the

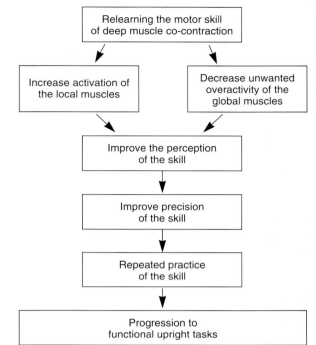

**Figure 7.4**    The elements of relearning the motor skill. (Based on Kottke et al.[196])

global muscles do not contribute to the task. These principles are at the very heart of learning a skill and, therefore, form the basis of the exercise programme to re-establish segmental stability of the spine. The essential elements of learning a new skill are outlined in Figure 7.4. The principles were first documented by Kottke et al[196] and have been applied in varying fields of practice by a number of other researchers and clinicians.[2,305]

These principles for relearning a motor skill were utilized by Hides et al[136] and O'Sullivan et al[257,259] in their clinical trials of efficacy of this specific exercise approach for segmental stabilization training. They used the methods of gaining the perception of the skill and repeated practice to achieve their successful outcomes and fulfil their aim to rehabilitate the development of the motor skill linked to deep muscle co-contraction. Initial evidence that skill training can change an automatic pattern of abdominal muscle activity in response to an unilateral arm-raising task has been reported by O'Sullivan et al,[259] in addition to our preliminary results of three patients with low back pain. These latter patients were evaluated using EMG with fine-wire electrodes before and after implementation of training of the transversus abdominis using the approach defined here. They were shown to attain earlier contraction of the transversus abdominis in the limb-movement task (see Ch. 4) following treatment (G.A. Jull & Q. Scott, unpublished data 1998).

## THE APPROACH TO CLINICAL TESTING

The clinical test of the deep muscle co-contraction is not performed in a functional upright position but in prone lying. The relationship between the wanted and unwanted muscle activity in perfecting a motor skill helps clarify why the clinical motor skill test of abdominal drawing in, in the prone position (see Ch. 8), has proven to be successful in identifying and checking the action of the transversus abdominis and lumbar multifidus. The prone position allows a more focused testing procedure by decreasing the need to use the larger global abdominal muscles to hold body position, as would occur in upright positions. In the prone position, activation of the transversus abdominis, by drawing in the abdominal wall without movement of the spine or pelvis, should be achieved with minimal activation of the global muscles that link the rib cage and the pelvis when its independent motor control is operating effectively. In the low back pain patient, monitoring of the levels of unwanted muscle activity can also be a feature of the test.

The requirements of the clinical motor skill test to hold a tonic, smoothly generated, isometric contraction without phasic, jerky contractions is also warranted in the light of another feature of the motor control problems found in the transversus abdominis of back pain patients. Back pain patients demonstrated phasic activity with arm movement instead of the normal tonic activity. A slowly generated 10-s hold should test this aspect of motor control (see Ch. 6). In relation to therapeutics, Hides et al[136] in their clinical trial used an isometric (tonic) hold of the segmental lumbar multifidus to restore its cross-sectional area following its inhibition with an acute episode of back pain. Recovery did not occur with the resumption of normal activities in the control group, despite resolution of the pain. O'Sullivan et al[257,259] used similar isometric holding exercises in their successful treatment of patients with low back pain associated with segmental instability.

Recently, more detailed observations in our clinical laboratory are providing preliminary evidence that drawing in of the abdominal wall in normal subjects usually results in the automatic activation of the lumbar multifidus. In addition, the relationship between activation of the pelvic floor and the activation of the transversus abdominis has been readily observed (see Ch. 9). The observed co-activation of the transversus abdominis and lumbar multifidus may well represent the way in which these muscles are controlled to provide lumbopelvic support during movement, and is a key factor in the clinical tests and their interpretation. For example, subjects who, while attempting the drawing-in test, do not co-activate the multifidus, or those achieving the multifidus activation test without co-activation of the transversus abdominis, could be demonstrating a significant deficit in one aspect of motor control. More research is required to verify these observations.

## REHABILITATION APPROACH

To provide joint stabilization, the nervous system needs to plan to recruit as well as maintain control of the motor units within the large numbers of muscles capable of influencing lumbopelvic position. For segmental control, it is the way the motor units of the local and deep system of muscles are recruited and their activation continuously modulated which is the essence of the rehabilitation process. The motor-control deficit in the activation patterns is patient specific, often complex and likely to involve problems in both the feedback and feedforward mechanisms of motor control.

Rehabilitation takes place in three distinct stages: formal motor skill training; gradual incorporation of skill into light functional tasks; and progression to heavy-load functional tasks. In this way, rehabilitation of the muscle system proceeds from control at the segmental level to control of the entire lumbopelvic region and trunk during the performance of functional tasks. At all stages of rehabilitation other treatments also need to be directed towards eliminating the influences of pain or reflex inhibition on muscle function.

## Formal motor skill training

Restoration of the motor skill of a drawing in of the abdominal wall with an isometric contraction of the lumbar multifidus is a consistent central point of the rehabilitation programme. Formal training of this motor skill to activate the deep muscles in their supporting role is approached by following the established principles for skill acquisition and relearning of a motor skill (see Fig. 7.4). Key components include the development of the perception of the skill and improving the precision. This is followed by the precise repetition of that skill in order for it to become automatically incorporated into normal function. Progression from this formal training stage is commensurate with cognitive control of this motor skill, which needs to be tested clinically in the prone test with some quantification from the pressure biofeedback unit (see Ch. 8).

### Development of the perception of the specific contraction of the local muscles

There are several reasons why it is essential for a back pain patient to develop the correct perception of, and achieve, the isolated muscle actions inherent in the motor skill of drawing in the abdominal wall as well as to learn the feeling of a tonic holding contraction of the deep local muscle system. These reasons are directly related to the research evidence of the nature of the motor control deficits in the deep muscles. As described previously, the transversus abdominis

has a separate control system. It is activated prior to the other trunk muscles involved in general trunk postural control and its pre-programmed activity is not direction specific (see Ch. 4). The opposite occurs in back pain patients (see Ch. 5). The muscle becomes controlled with postural control and becomes direction specific, behaving as if it were part of the global muscle system of the abdominal wall. It loses its functional identification to prepare the spinal segment for loads and forces imposed by general activities. A focus on training the specific motor skill by isolating the contraction as much as possible from the other abdominal muscles aims to restore normal motor commands for the muscle (cognitively in the first instance). The need to focus or isolate the contraction of the lumbar multifidus to a segmental level relates to its primary segmental site of dysfunction[136,139] as well as its functional differentiation from the other trunk extensors[37] and the segmental lack of response to general activity of the trunk extensors in normal activity.[136] In addition to an ability to isolate the deep muscle contraction, it is necessary for the patient to be able to perceive slow continuous muscle activity as the deep muscles lose their ability to hold tonically in back pain patients.

In management, different patients will respond to different strategies in the relearning process to achieve the motor skill of deep muscle co-activation. The clinician must be prepared to try different strategies, often in combination, until one which works for the individual patient is found. The following are suggestions that can be tried to enhance the patient's perception of the deep muscle motor skill:

- Focus on one particular muscle (of the local system) at a time.
- Try different instructions, visual cues or mental imagery.
- Try different postures and positions.
- Use various forms of facilitation and feedback techniques to increase deep muscle activation.
- Use various techniques (including feedback) to decrease overactivity of the global muscles during the deep muscle isolation exercises.

*Precise repetition of the correct isolated holding action of the deep muscles in a co-activation pattern*

Repeated practice of the correct motor skill of abdominal drawing in with lumbar multifidus activation is vital for learning and for training the deep muscle co-activation. In addition, the focus on continuous holding is commensurate with the type of muscle contraction required for stabilization. Lack of this tonic function is a problem in the deep muscles of low back pain patients, and training of this continuous holding contraction has been linked to successful management of both acute and chronic low back pain patients.[136,257,259]

Repetitions are performed precisely using the focus, the cues, the positions and other techniques found successful in isolating the deep muscle action. This will likely be different for each individual patient. It is essential that the therapist provides appropriate instruction and cues to ensure that the patient will practise the skill correctly at home. Motivation to practise the motor skill as many times as possible is the key to this part of the rehabilitation. Progression to more functional tasks can be begun once the assessment has demonstrated that the motor skill has been learned.

## Integration into dynamic function

The exercise approach integrating deep muscle co-contraction into dynamic function proceeds through two stages: incorporation of the motor skill into light functional tasks, and incorporation of the skill into heavy loaded tasks. The use of light functional tasks in the first instance allows deep muscle support to be trained during activities where the global muscles are moving the lumbopelvic region. In contrast, heavy activities require all trunk muscles (local and global) to contract simultaneously in order to brace and stabilize the torso to resist the external loads, and require a different type of functional training.

It is necessary to have ways to ensure that deep muscle action is being maintained during the integration of the motor skill into dynamic function. Methods include:

- Instruct the patient to activate the co-contraction cognitively during all exercise tasks.
- Formally retest the co-contraction at regular intervals.
- Indirectly assess the transversus abdominis contraction by observing the abdominal wall. The abdominal wall should remain flat with no protrusion or bulging (particularly of the lower abdomen) during any exercise.[242]
- Indirectly assess multifidus function through observing the patient's ability to maintain the normal lumbosacral curve during any exercise.[22]

*Incorporation of motor skill into light functional tasks*

This stage involves continued practice of the motor skill in low-load tasks during which relaxed breathing can continue normally without breath-holding. The progression to training in light functional tasks continues a focus on the rehabilitation of the motor control of the deep trunk muscles in concert with their stability synergists, the diaphragm and the pelvic floor. It is in these light-load activities, especially in neutral postures, that the lumbar segments particularly require the support of the local muscle system.[54] Therefore, this training phase starts in the neutral lumbopelvic postural positions where maximum local muscle activation is required to control spinal position. Varying tasks are gradually added which increasingly challenge the function of the deep muscle system.

*Control of neutral lumbopelvic postures*

A variety of activities is used for training the holding of the deep muscles in functional activities. In the first instance, assuming and holding good upright sitting and standing postures with the lumbopelvic region in a neutral posture and with co-activation of the deep muscles is a potent, patient-convenient and functionally relevant training regime. Turning, reaching and leaning slightly away from the neutral positions, all with normal relaxed breathing patterns, further challenge control of the deep muscle system.[124] The ability to maintain the control of the spinal position under low levels of leg load can also be trained.[176,294,295]

The efficiency of the methods chosen to improve transversus abdominis and lumbar multifidus activation and holding capacity should be continually checked in the formal prone test using pressure biofeedback. Assessment in these functional tasks by means of observation and palpation only does not give a reliable indication of the improvement in deep muscle capacity.

### Lumbopelvic control during trunk movements

Walking offers an excellent functional activity to challenge and advance the training of the motor skill of holding the deep muscle co-activation for segmental support and control. It requires quite complex motor planning. Walking is a phasic, repetitive, low-load activity which provides a situation that requires the patient to maintain tonic control of the local muscles in an environment requiring phasic on/off activation from the larger global trunk muscles. Precision and a good perception of the contraction is required by the patient, who activates the deep muscle system either by holding the gentle abdominal drawing-in action or through activating and holding a pelvic floor muscle contraction while breathing normally. This type of functional activity would likely optimize the stabilizing capabilities of the deep muscles. Training can be advanced by increasing the length of time for which the patient holds the contraction and increasing the speed of walking. Notably, the phasic on/off patterns of trunk muscle activity are the antithesis of the continuous tonic activity required of the deep local muscle system in its supporting role (see Ch. 6). Again, assurance that the training is beneficial and not detrimental to the deep muscle system is gained by repeatedly assessing the patient's performance in the prone position.

### Lumbopelvic control in aggravating postures

The deep muscle co-contraction is also trained in spinal postural positions which normally aggravate the patient's pain, and in postures where patients report that their backs feel vulnerable and likely to 'give'.[257] Patients can train in the static aggravating posture, such as sitting, or in other upright functional activities, such as walking. They may also formally train to maintain the co-contraction while moving their trunk through movement directions that usually aggravate their pain.

## Incorporation of skill into heavy-load functional tasks

Everyday function incorporates coping with activities involving higher external loads, as in lifting and carrying, as well as in activities such as stepping down or jumping in which the local and global systems of both the trunk and lower limbs work together to minimize impact loading to the spine. Therapeutic exercise in higher load activities can be advanced with two different treatment aims in mind.

With the first aim, exercise focuses on ensuring that the deep local muscles remain the functional stabilizers of the lumbopelvic region even when higher load activities are attempted. The more general stabilization training programmes still maintain neutral lumbopelvic postures and train more general trunk muscle co-contraction on both stable and unstable surfaces. The focus of these exercises is on control of spinal position rather than the resistance force.[101,176,188,288,293–295,353] It is still important to emphasize the action of the transversus abdominis and lumbar multifidus during such activities. It is of interest that Thompson[331] has calculated that the transversus abdominis is the abdominal muscle which is exposed to the most stress loading during lifting activities.

The second aim relates to assessing and treating any dysfunction in the muscles of the global system. Strength, endurance and coordination are required in the larger muscles of the lower limb, pelvis and trunk to cope with impact loading inherent in daily activities. In addition, any overactivity and restrictions caused by the multijoint muscles in the lumbopelvic hip complex[163,173] may need to be addressed in the total therapeutic exercise programme.

As a general statement, progression to higher load activities could begin as soon as the healing of the injured tissue allows, providing that this high-level training does not compromise the specific motor relearning programme for the transversus abdominis and lumbar multifidus. As an example, if global muscles such as the obliquus externus abdominis are found to be overactive in tests of the specific motor skill of deep muscle co-activation and techniques to decrease their activity are being employed in the motor skill reeducation, then it would certainly be unwise to begin the progression to higher load training. Such training focuses on the global muscle system and could reinforce, or even increase, the patient's deep muscle motor control problems.

At every stage of the rehabilitation it is necessary to come back to the formal test of the deep muscle motor skill to ensure that the co-activation is maintaining or improving its level of activation and tonic holding capacity. During the progression to heavy functional loading of the trunk, it is also essential to monitor improvements and to guide progression of these stages. Sophisticated apparatus is available to measure trunk muscle strength and endurance in each plane of motion,[268] and functional lifting capacity assessments are also well documented.[161] How-

ever, formal measures of improvement in general trunk stability capacity as a result of the more general stabilization training programmes are not as well documented, as trunk co-contraction is not an easy function to measure. One way of gaining an assessment is through the use of the leg-loading tests with pressure biofeedback (see Ch. 8).

Rehabilitation has progressed from new concepts of retraining the deep muscles to incorporation of these concepts into normal function. The essence of the treatment is that the supporting function of the deep muscles, working in co-contraction to control segmental movement, is restored. Increasing general trunk stiffness through increased co-contraction of the global muscles, which could encourage some trunk rigidity, is not considered a reasonable aim of treatment unless deep muscle function has been severely compromised. There are differences between segmental stability provided by the transversus abdominis and lumbar multifidus and lumbar rigidity provided by strong contraction of the global muscles. The transversus abdominis and lumbar multifidus offer control segmentally and allow trunk movement to occur in a controlled manner. In contrast, the global muscles restrict motion of the spine, promoting function of the trunk as a single entity. Normal function of the spine relies on controlled motion of the lumbar segments and not general restriction of motion. In Section 4 the details of the new assessment and treatment approach for low back pain patients are explained.

# The clinical approach

A high level of skill is required to effectively rehabilitate the motor control changes present in low back pain patients. In addition, skill is required to effectively communicate 'spinal segmental training' to a patient and a considerable amount of practice required for the therapist to achieve the necessary level of competence. For this reason the description of the exercise approach is presented here in considerable detail. Therapists need to take time to develop their problem solving and assessment skills of the motor control problems in back pain patients. Success in treatment is always closely aligned to the diagnostic and therapeutic skills of the practitioner.

# 8

# Clinical testing of the local muscles: practical examination of motor skill

The use of evidence-based treatments is the call of the decade and the practice for the 21st century. With this new insight into the muscle problems associated with low back pain, assessment and measurement of the impairment must take priority. While invasive methods of verifying motor control problems in the deep muscle exist (see Ch. 5), there is an immediate priority to investigate non-invasive clinically applicable measures of motor control deficits. Developing clinically feasible measurements for this aspect of muscle function is an essential challenge to physiotherapists. Beckerman et al[30] highlight the challenges of measurement development in their recent review of the efficacy of physiotherapy treatments and the inherent problems found in most published clinical research studies. These authors emphasize that evaluation is the key to proving efficacy of treatments. However, they also acknowledge that there is a lack of physical outcome parameters that are valid, precise, sensitive and clinically relevant.

It must be acknowledged that measurement of motor-control problems will always present difficulties in both the clinic and in research, in comparison to such measures as strength and endurance of muscle groups. Additional challenges present in low back pain patients. The muscles exhibiting the deficits are those which lie deep in the body and close to the spine. Their location means that their contraction cannot be viewed from the surface of the body. The muscles are not involved in movement of the bony skeleton, and traditional muscle testing procedures such as manual muscle testing, which rely on movement of the skeletal lever system, do not apply. While it will be a significant length of time before the non-invasive assessments of the motor control deficits in deep muscles have reached gold standards, some progress has been made.

Traditional muscle-function measures of strength and endurance of muscle groups or cardiovascular endurance routinely involve a period of practice in which the motor skills are learnt and the body systems adjust to the task. The measures become reliable and repeatable as the learning phase is replaced quite quickly with a 'levelling out' of the performance. Standard levels can then be readily quantified. Improvement in the performance of these muscle functions takes time. The body systems need adequate stimulus and time to demonstrate a change in the measures.

A far more difficult task is presented when developing measurements of a motor skill such as the isometric, continuous low level contraction of the local muscles, which is performed independently of any contribution from the global muscles. The measurement must further cope with a confounding variable of possible unwanted overactivity in these global muscles. In contrast to the measurements of strength or endurance of muscle groups, issues of repeatability and reliability become quite challenging factors in cases of disordered motor control. For example, during the learning phase, improvement can occur immediately and the measures change on repeated assessments if the patient develops the perception of the isolated contraction quickly. Other patients with possibly more severe deficits may take days or even weeks to understand and learn the perception of the contraction. Such patients can often be identified on the factor of variability which disturbs the

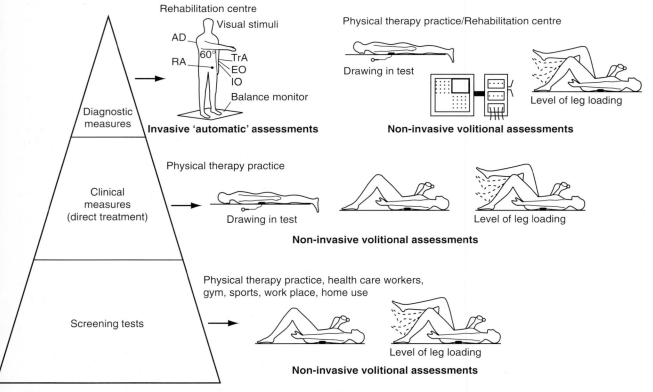

**Figure 8.1** The three-tier model for assessing deep muscle dysfunction. AD, anterior deltoid; OE, obliquus externus abdominis; OI, obliquus internus abdominis; RA, rectus abdominis; TrA, transversus abdominis.

traditional model of baseline repeatability. This poses challenges and difficulties for measurement which, to a large extent, are being overcome through the clinical research currently being undertaken in our laboratory.

## MODEL OF ASSESSMENT

A three-tier model of assessment is proposed at the present time to assess the degree of motor control deficit in the local muscle system of the lumbopelvic region (Fig. 8.1). This model is tiered in degrees of sophistication of the assessment and, accordingly, the depth, type and detail of information that can be derived. In parallel, the complexity of the measure used increases from first to third tier: screening tests, clinical assessments and diagnostic assessments.

The first tier is a simple measure and is comparatively crude. It is a non-invasive volitional test and is based on the clinical assessment of the abdominal drawing-in action while controlling lumbopelvic posture during progressive leg loading. The use of the pressure biofeedback unit provides some quantification for this test (see the Appendix to this chapter for a description of the biofeedback unit). This test provides a means of assessing whether or not the deep muscles are working with the contraction of the global muscles, but does not measure specific details of the motor control deficits. As such, it is suitable as a screening measure and is useful not only for physical therapists but also for general use by healthcare workers or exercise trainers in workplaces and gymnasiums or for individual home use. As back pain is a very common and costly condition, this level of testing may potentially be important with respect to the prevention and management of non-complex low back pain. Research is needed to validate these testing methods when performed by personnel who are unfamiliar with the motor control problems of the deep muscles and their treatment.

The second-tier clinical assessments are detailed non-invasive volitional tests that have been devised to give an indication of the normal function of the deep muscles. Use is made not only of the pressure biofeedback, but also of electromyographic biofeedback and observation of the body contours and breathing patterns in order to detect the deficits in deep muscle activation. These assessments require the clinical knowledge and skill of a physical therapist and are used to direct treatment strategies (see Ch. 9).

The third tier includes two potentially diagnostic assessment measures of deep muscle function. One uses electromyography (EMG) with fine-wire electrodes inserted into the deep muscles in order to measure directly the degree of motor-control deficit in a reaction time task. This measure does not rely on patient volition and is being developed from the research model described in Chapters 4 and 5. The second measure is a non-invasive volitional assessment using a combination of ultrasound imaging, measures from a pressure sensor and surface EMG. This measure is currently being developed not only for diagnosing the motor control deficits in the deep muscles but also to direct and evaluate more precisely the re-education strategies.

In this book, emphasis is placed on the second-tier clinical assessments for the recognition of the deficits in the transversus abdominis and lumbar multifidus. A detailed description of the leg-loading tests used to assess control of lumbopelvic posture is also included. These are used in clinical assessments, and also form the basis of the screening tests.

## CLINICAL ASSESSMENT

The clinical assessment of the deep muscle co-contraction involves: the abdominal drawing-in test, the segmental multifidus test and the leg-loading test. The transversus abdominis and the lumbar multifidus are tested separately initially, as one or the other, or both, may demonstrate impairments in low back pain patients.

### Testing the tranversus abdominis: the abdominal drawing-in test

The prone abdominal drawing-in test measures a level of motor skill competence, i.e. it measures

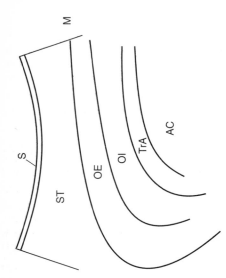

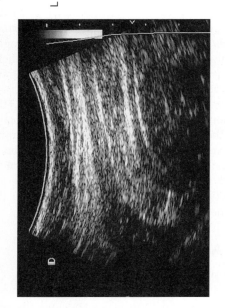

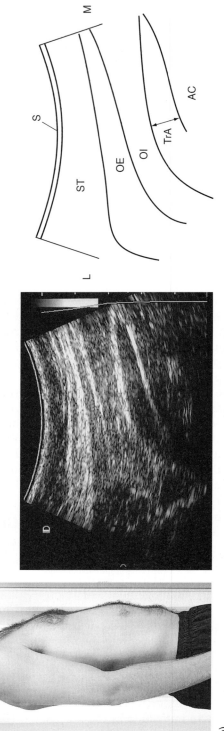

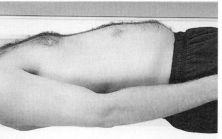

(a)

(b)

**Figure 8.2** The action of transversus abdominis: (a) the relaxed abdominal wall; (b) the drawn-in abdominal wall. The ultrasound images are of a transverse section of the abdominal wall. The shape and width of the transversus abdominis (TrA) can be seen to change on contraction (the width has increased (↔)), with little change in the obliquus externus abdominis (OE) and obliquus internus abdominis (OI). AC, abdominal contents; L, lateral; M, medial; S, skin; ST, subcutaneous tissue.

the ability of the patient to use the correct muscles (mainly the transversus abdominis and lumbar multifidus) in response to the command 'Draw in your abdominal wall without moving your spine or pelvis and hold for 10 s while breathing normally'. There is also the requirement to perform this action without the contraction of the global muscles.

*Teaching the action in preparation for the test*

**Principle.**   The motor skill under examination is not a familiar task to the patient, and teaching the action well is an integral part of the assessment procedure. The action of the transversus abdominis is to draw in the abdominal wall and narrow the waist. Thus the principle underlying the teaching of the contraction is to instruct the patient to draw in the abdominal wall in a way which produces contraction of the transversus abdominis in isolation from the other abdominal muscles. The most successful way to achieve this is to instruct the patient to concentrate on the lower part of the abdomen. Additional recent evidence suggests that the lower portion of the transversus abdominis may be the part most essential for spinal stabilization.[144]

The drawing in of the lower abdomen is illustrated in Figure 8.2. The ultrasound images of the anterolateral aspect of abdominal wall just superior to the iliac crest show the muscle at rest and following the performance of drawing in of the lower abdomen. Note the increase in width of the transversus abdominis, and the minimal change in the obliquus externus abdominis and internus. An important feature of this view of the transversus abdominis is its circular, corset-like shape when it is contracted, drawing in the waist.

**Describing the task.**   Due to the precision required for the accurate performance of the test of transversus abdominis function, it is essential for the patient to have a good picture of the muscle together with a knowledge of the required contraction. A description of the basic anatomy of the muscle, an illustration of the muscle (Fig. 8.3) and the movement required are

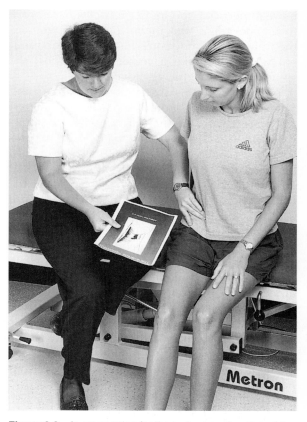

**Figure 8.3**   In preparation for the test, an explanation of the anatomy of the transversus abdominis assists the patient in understanding the direction of the muscle contraction.

helpful tools. A good analogy to use in teaching is to describe the transversus abdominis as the patient's own natural deep muscle 'corset' that surrounds the abdomen in the same way as an external corset. When it contracts it draws in to tighten like an external corset to protect the back from injury. Instruction about the basic anatomy of the other abdominal muscles (the rectus abdominis, obliquus externus abdominis and internus abdominis) also highlights the difference between the transversus abdominis and other abdominal muscles, and assists the patient to make the distinction between movement of the trunk and abdominal drawing in. These muscles run from the pelvis to the rib cage without attachment to the lumbar vertebrae. The patient should understand that the job of the more superficial abdominal muscles is to work to tilt the pelvis and move the trunk, whereas the transversus abdominis narrows the abdominal wall to act like a corset and support the spine without producing movement.

Together with this description of anatomy and function, emphasis should be placed on the need for precision rather than effort. Many patients will find it difficult to understand the importance of isolation rather than strength. This can be overcome by drawing from research and describing the importance of the timing of the contraction of this muscle. In normal function it contracts prior to the other trunk muscles to help prepare the spinal joints for the forces of the activity, whereas in people with low back pain contraction is delayed. An explanation can be given of the deleterious effects on the injured and painful lumbar segment if the muscle contracts too late, regardless of how strong it is, or if the muscle cannot hold in a continuous manner during function. A description of the problems can help the patient to appreciate what is being achieved by testing in this manner.

**Instruction.** Instruction of the contraction involves a description of drawing up and in of the lower part of the abdomen towards the spine without movement of the trunk or pelvis, thus allowing the transversus abdominis to contract by itself without substitution by the other abdominal muscles. Additional assistance can be provided by the clinician placing his or her hands on their own abdomen and demonstrating the movement of the lower abdomen towards the spine. Demonstration of the action by the clinician with movement of their own abdomen is helpful. In the initial stages it is best to instruct the patient in the basics rather than to focus on trying to avoid or indeed correct all the possible substitution strategies (see Ch. 9). This approach also allows for a more standard testing protocol. These basics are to avoid movement of the trunk and pelvis, to keep the spine in a steady position and to avoid deep inspiration to simulate the abdominal wall movement.

The four-point kneeling position is an easy position in which to teach the patient the action in the first instance prior to formal testing (Fig. 8.4). This position permits increased awareness of the abdominal wall due to the gravitational stretch on the muscles, and allows complete relaxation of the abdominal wall, which is difficult in other positions such as standing.[83] In four-point kneeling with a relaxed abdomen the transversus abdominis is more in its lengthened position, which increases the range of muscle movement during the contraction, which in turn

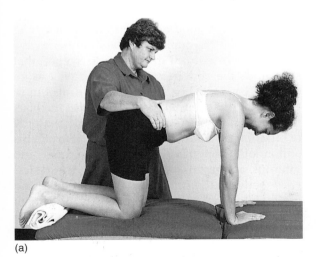

(a)                                             (b)

**Figure 8.4** Teaching the test action in the four-point kneeling position: (a) with the abdomen relaxed; (b) following the abdominal drawing-in action. Note the elevation of the lower abdominal wall.

increases the patient's awareness of the task being performed. Finally, the load of the abdominal contents and the length of the muscle in this position may increase the sensitivity of the stretch receptors, making it easier to contract the muscle. As a clinical note, while four-point kneeling is a good position for initial teaching of the action, it may not be a suitable treatment position for patients who have problems relaxing their abdominal wall and exhibit overactivity in their global muscles.

The first step is to ensure that the subject is relaxed in the four-point kneeling position. The hips should be over the knees and the shoulders directly over the hands, with the elbows relaxed and not forced into extension. The spine should be in a neutral position, although correction of the spinal position should be uncomplicated at this stage so that the patient can concentrate on the abdominal contraction. It is important to instruct the patient to relax the abdomen. The action performed is a drawing up and in of the lower abdomen with the instruction to take a relaxed breath in and out and then, without breathing in, draw the abdomen up towards the spine without taking a breath. It is essential to dissociate breathing from the performance of the contraction since the patient may simulate the abdominal movement simply by reducing the pressure in the thorax, drawing the diaphragm up and the abdominal wall in, in the same manner as when a person breathes in to squeeze through a narrow space. The contraction must be performed in a slow and controlled manner, and this should be emphasized from the beginning. Any motion of the spine and pelvis should be discouraged as soon as it is observed, as the test relies on a steady spine position.

Once the contraction has been achieved the patient should commence breathing in a slow and controlled manner, holding the contraction for 10 s. If it is difficult for a patient to breathe in this manner, and he or she substitutes rapid and shallow upper chest breathing, it should be noted, as this gives an indication that the patient may not be able to do the formal test correctly. At the completion of the task the contraction should be released in a slow and controlled

manner. Patients should perform the task several times to achieve sufficient proficiency of the contraction to allow accurate objective testing. However, the clinician should bear in mind that fatigue has a significant influence on the contraction of the transversus abdominis. Fatigue can generally be identified as either deterioration in performance, increased substitution or tremor. Occasionally, patients will become frustrated because the task they are being asked to perform seems impossible due to the required precision. The clinician should be aware of this and be understanding, allowing the patient sufficient time to absorb the information. Finally, the clinician should emphasize again that the test is one of control and precision, not strength.

### The formal test

Once the action is understood by the patient, the formal test is conducted in prone lying, using a pressure biofeedback unit (see Appendix) to obtain a measurement of the ability of the patient to perform this abdominal isolation test (Fig. 8.5). Isolated contraction of the transversus abdominis is more difficult in the prone position, because this position eliminates some of the stimuli present in the four-point kneeling position. This helps to distinguish between people

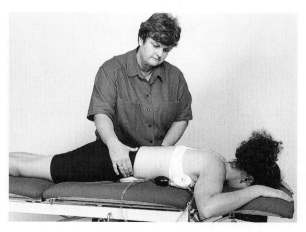

**Figure 8.5**    The abdominal drawing-in test in the prone position. (Note: The arm is flexed so that the position of the biofeedback unit can be seen.)

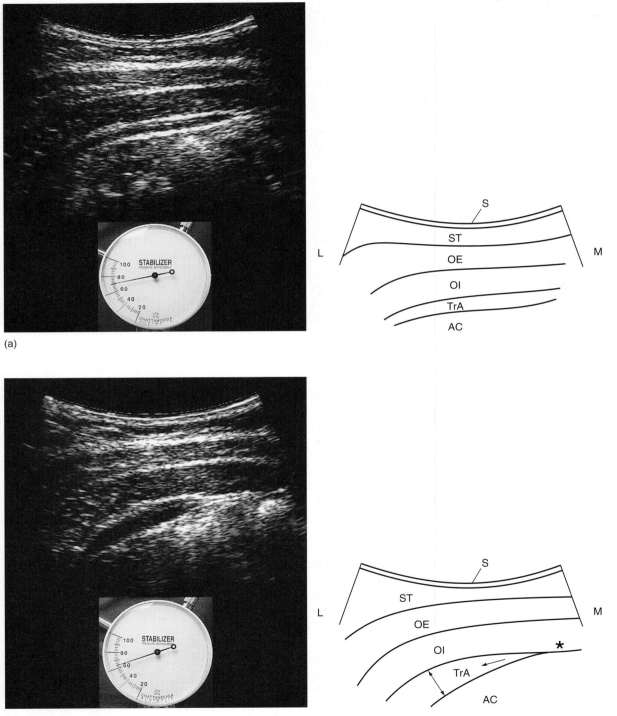

(a)

(b)

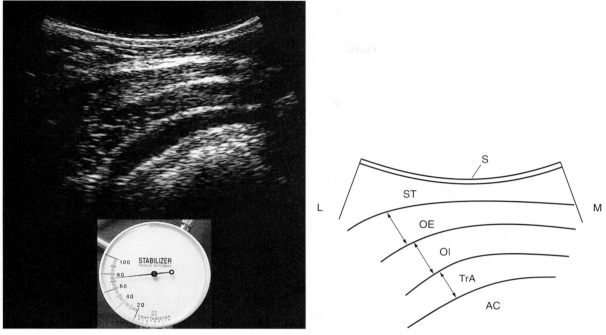

(c)

**Figure 8.6**    The pressure changes seen using the biofeedback unit and ultrasound images (transverse section of the anterolateral abdominal wall) recorded during the clinical abdominal drawing-in test. (a) At rest before the test; the baseline pressure is 70 mmHg. (b) On correct performance of the abdominal drawing-in action. The pressure reduces by 6–10 mmHg. The contraction of the transversus abdominis (TrA) can be seen on the ultrasound image. Note the corset-like appearance and the tensioning on the fascia medially (*). On contraction, the width of the TrA increases. (c) On incorrect performance of the abdominal drawing-in action, the pressure is increased slightly. The ultrasound image shows contraction of all the muscles of the abdominal wall simultaneously. The obliquus externus abdominis (OE), obliquus internus abdominis (OI), have contracted together and each has increased in depth (↔). There is no corset action of the TrA. AC, abdominal contents; L, lateral; M, medial; S, skin; ST, subcutaneous tissue.

who can perform the test poorly and those who can perform it well. The patient lies prone with the arms by the side, and the pressure biofeedback unit is placed under the abdomen with the navel in the centre and the distal edge of the pad in line with the right and left anterior superior iliac spines. The pressure pad is inflated to 70 mmHg and allowed to stabilize. This pressure has been identified to be that which inflates the pad sufficiently to detect changes in position of the abdominal wall but is comfortable and does not press into the abdominal contents. At rest, small deviations of the indicator on the pressure dial will be evident with abdominal movement during normal respiration, and thus it is essential to identify the point about which the level fluctuates.

The muscle contraction in the formal test of the motor skill is identical to that performed in the four-point kneeling position, although the emphasis in instruction may be changed to drawing in the abdomen to support the weight of the abdominal contents off the pad. The instructions are again to breathe in and out and then, without breathing in, to slowly draw in the abdomen so that it lifts up off the pad, keeping the spinal position steady. Deep inspiration is to be avoided, as is any movement of the pelvis and trunk. Once the contraction has been achieved the patient should recommence relaxed normal breathing. The test action can be repeated until the clinician is confident that the contraction is being performed as optimally as possible by the patient. Once satisfied, the action is repeated and the pressure change noted. The patient is required to hold the contraction for 10 s. The procedure can be repeated up to 10 times to test the endurance of the muscles.

**Test results.** The pressure biofeedback unit provides important information about the relationship between the local and global muscles of the anterior abdominal wall. A successful performance of the test reduces the pressure by 6–10 mmHg. This pressure change indicates that the patient is able to contract the transversus abdominis into its shortened range, independently of the other abdominal muscles (Fig. 8.6a,b,c). If the patient can successfully reduce the pressure in this test, then the holding capacity of the contraction is tested through repetition of 10-s holds up to a maximum of 10 repeats.

In this stage of testing, it is essential to ensure that the patient has not simply tilted the pelvis or flexed the spine to reduce the pressure, which would give a false-positive test response. A drop of less than 2 mmHg, no change in pressure or an increase in pressure is a poor result, and indicates that the patient is unable to contract the transversus abdominis into its shortened range independently of the other abdominal muscles. The failure to drop the pressure by the required amount may relate to one of two factors: the inability to activate the transversus abdominis to a sufficient level; or the contraction of the global muscles, which act to flatten (rather than narrow) the waist due to their longitudinal attachment from the pelvis to the rib cage, in conjunction with the transversus abdominis. A pressure increase often occurs if the patient is substituting for the contraction of transversus abdominis by contraction of the rectus abdominis or obliquus externus abdominis. The latter are superficial muscles and, as they contract, they push on the pad (see Fig. 8.6c). EMG surface electrodes can be placed on the likely overactive global muscles (i.e. the obliquus externus abdominis or rectus abdominis) to give an additional means of quantifying their overactivity. The full analysis of the poor test result

acts as a basis for selecting the most suitable treatment strategies, and is described fully in Chapter 9.

**Note on testing.** Many people with low back pain will find it very difficult to gain a perception of the required contraction and will demonstrate a poor test result. Some people with no history of low back pain may also have difficulty in gaining this perception and may need some degree of skill training to perform the contraction, although this will always be much less than that required by back pain sufferers. This fact emphasizes two points: the need for a good level of clinical skill in order to teach the person, and the need to employ some facilitation strategies in the initial phases of teaching.

It may be impractical to perform the test in the prone position in obese patients, in those with impaired lumbar spine mobility or patients with significant respiratory disease. In these cases, the abdominal drawing-in action can be assessed in either supine lying or by observation of the abdominal wall in four-point kneeling, standing or supported standing. Nevertheless, it must be realized that these visual assessments do not give reliable information about the performance of the transversus abdominis.

### Relationship between low back pain and the test

Several studies have been undertaken to evaluate whether the ability to perform the clinical test of transversus abdominis function can identify people with low back pain. The first of these involved the assessment of 37 people presenting to a medical practice for problems other than low back pain.[282] Fifty-four percent of the subjects had a history of low back pain. The examiners were blinded to the presentation of the subjects. Subjects undertook the abdominal drawing-in test in the prone position, and the examiner recorded any pressure reduction. Using the criterion that a drop of less than 6 mmHg or an increase in pressure indicates poor transversus abdominis activation, the examiners could correctly classify 90% of subjects as having a history of low back pain.

The second study involved the assessment by a blinded examiner of a group of eight low back pain patients and 14 control subjects with no history of low back pain.[175] In this study the ability to reduce the pressure was noted, and EMG recordings were made of the rectus abdominis, obliquus externus abdominis and obliquus internus abdominis. Again a significant difference was found between the groups in terms of their ability to reduce pressure in the sensor (subjects with low back pain were essentially unable to do so). The reasons for this difference in pressure change were difficult to determine in this study. The patients with low back pain did have significantly greater use of the lower portion of their rectus abdominis, with no change in the oblique muscles. Unfortunately, the transversus abdominis, the muscle responsible for drawing in the abdominal wall, was not assessed. However, this study does draw our attention to the level of operator skill required in assessments, as well as the need for future studies to include fine-wire EMG to measure the contraction of the transversus abdominis.

### Relationship between clinical and laboratory tests

An important question is whether the delayed contraction of the transversus abdominis in people with low back pain, as determined in laboratory motor control studies, is related to the clinical tests of the ability to perform an isolated contraction of this muscle. This question was assessed in a study in which subjects with and without low back pain were assessed using the clinical test and by evaluation of the timing of onset of contraction of the transversus abdominis in a limb-movement task.[153] In this study subjects were classified into poor function, good function and intermediate groups on the basis of their ability to reduce pressure and the time of onset of electromyographic activity. Although the measures were not correlated, there was good agreement between those subjects with a poor ability to decrease the pressure and those with a delay in transversus abdominis contraction, and between subjects who could

decrease the pressure and those who had early activation of transversus abdominis. Thus, the quality of motor control of the transversus abdominis, which can be measured directly only by using indwelling electrodes (which are not readily available in clinical practice), can be estimated indirectly from the performance shown in the clinical assessments.

## Testing the segmental lumbar multifidus

Screening assessments of the segmental lumbar multifidus are difficult for unskilled testers, as they rely on sensitive palpation. However, the experienced clinician can make a clinical judgement through palpation of the muscle contraction at the segmental level. The clinical assessment of the lumbar multifidus is conducted in the prone position, as in the abdominal drawing-in test. While it would be expected that the lumbar multifidus would contract together with the transversus abdominis in the prone position test, specific commands and techniques are used to better focus the concentration of the clinician and patient on the lumbar multifidus, in order to test its activation and tonic holding ability separately at each segmental level.

Assessment of the lumbar multifidus begins with palpation of the muscle at each segment, with the patient relaxed and in the prone position (Fig. 8.7). The muscle is palpated adjacent to the spinous process and a side-to-side comparison

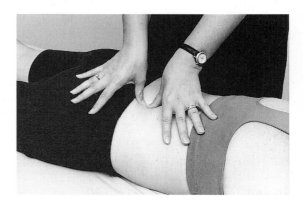

**Figure 8.7** Palpation for muscle consistency at adjacent vertebral levels.

is made at each lumbar level; in addition, a comparison is made of the segments above and below. The clinician feels for any loss in muscle consistency at the segment; this is in line with the segmental inhibition at the symptomatic segment detected by Hides et al [136] in their study of acute/subacute low back pain patients.

Like the test of the transversus abdominis, the test of the isolated activation of the lumbar multifidus at the segmental level can be considered as a specific motor skill. As indicated, the prone position test is used to measure a level of motor-skill competence. This test measures the ability of the patient to use the correct muscles (mainly the multifidus, with transversus abdominis) in response to the command 'Gently swell out your muscles under my fingers without moving your spine or pelvis. Hold the contraction while breathing normally'. There is no focus by the subject on the individual muscle actions, only on the tester's fingers gently compressing the muscle at a local segmental level and the instruction to swell out without spinal or pelvic movement. A variety of hand positions can be used to perform the test. The clinician can use the thumbs, the index or middle fingers of each hand, or the thumb and index fingers of one hand to palpate each segmental level. The fingers are gently but firmly sunk into the muscle belly in preparation for the test (Fig. 8.8). As for the test of the

transversus abdominis, the subject is asked to breathe in, then out, and to hold the breath out. The patient is instructed to gently and slowly swell out the muscle into the fingers, and to then resume normal breathing. The clinician concentrates on feeling for a deep development of tension in the muscle, which indicates the activation of multifidus at that segment. The patient's ability to hold the contraction indicates the muscle's tonic holding capacity. An inability to activate the segmental multifidus is indicated by palpating no or little muscle tension development under the fingers. A rapid and superficial development of tension is unsatisfactory, and indicates that either the patient is using only the superficial fibres in an extension action or the clinician is palpating the stiffness in the long tendons of the thoracic portion of erector spinae, which traverse the area. The action of these muscles instead of lumbar multifidus may also be observed directly by changes in the shape of the muscle bellies in the thoracic region. Alternatively, the amount of unnecessary muscle activity in these global muscles during the testing manoeuvre can be monitored using EMG. The other common strategy that the patient may use to simulate the correct action is a backward pelvic tilt, in an attempt to push the muscle back into the clinician's fingers.

The clinical assessment of the segmental lumbar multifidus is therefore made by the tester palpating the multifidus activation at each lumbar level, including whether a controlled tonic hold can be achieved. More objective evidence can be obtained through the use of real-time ultrasound imaging as the patient attempts the testing manoeuvre.[136] The depth of the multifidus changes during the isometric holding contraction, and this can be viewed using real-time ultrasound images. Figure 8.9 illustrates a longitudinal section of the multifidus at the L5 level when in a relaxed state (Fig. 8.9a) and when the muscle has contracted isometrically (Fig. 8.9b). An increase in depth of the muscle can be observed; this is the contraction measured by palpation of the segmental levels of the multifidus by the clinician.

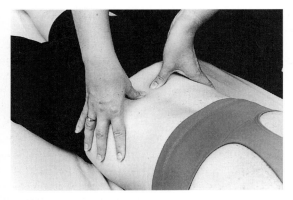

**Figure 8.8** Palpation for the contraction of the right and left muscles at each lumbar segment of the lumbar multifidus.

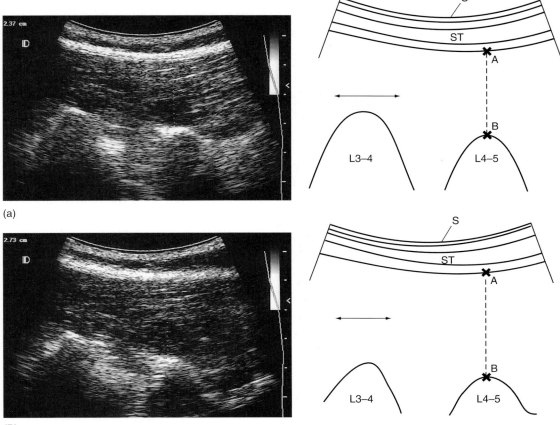

(a)

(B)

**Figure 8.9**    Ultrasound images of the lumbar multifidus in longitudinal section: (a) relaxed state; (b) after isometric contraction. The line AB represents the depth of the muscle from its superior aspect to the superior aspect of the L4–L5 zygapophyseal joint. In the relaxed state (a) this is 2.37 cm; on contraction (b), this depth increases to 2.73 cm. S, skin; ST subcutaneous tissue. The multifidus fibres run in the direction of the arrow ($\leftrightarrow$).

### *Relationship between clinical tests and other measures*

Real-time ultrasound imaging has been used to confirm both the palpation and activation tests for the multifidus. Imaging has been conducted formally for acute/subacute patients[136,139] and also informally in our research clinic. In acute/subacute low back pain patients, the changes in the muscle are specific to the affected vertebral level and to the symptomatic side in unilateral cases.[136,139] This localized response in the multifidus has been demonstrated using real-time ultrasound imaging and confirmed using mag-netic resonance imaging (MRI).[134] Furthermore, in 26 patients with acute/subacute low back pain, joints were examined manually to determine if the most affected vertebral level (as assessed by a blinded examiner) corresponded with the location of the changes in size of the multifidus. The results of the two independent tests corresponded in 24 of 26 cases.[139] The palpation test may be more difficult to perform in chronic low back pain patients, in whom changes such as disuse atrophy, fatty infiltration of muscle fibres, fibrosis and scar tissue may be present in the multifidus.

Real-time ultrasound imaging has been used to obtain objective evidence of the muscle contraction involved in the lumbar multifidus activation test.[136] The change in depth of the multifidus muscle, which the clinician palpates as a deep tensioning in the muscle, can be seen in the parasagittal section of the multifidus. The change in depth of the muscle from the relaxed to the contracted state can be seen in Figure 8.9.

Various patterns are emerging in the nature of multifidus muscle dysfunction in different patient groups, which we have been able to view using real-time ultrasound imaging. Acute low back pain patients commonly seem unable to activate the multifidus at the affected vertebral level. Chronic low back pain patients, on the other hand, exhibit different patterns. Some are unable to activate the multifidus, while others may perform quick, phasic contractions that are poorly controlled. Often there is a predominance of activity in the superficial fibres of the multifidus. With practice, the palpation test can be used by the clinician to detect these differences.

## Testing the control of lumbopelvic posture

We chose and developed a test model of leg loading in supine lying to quantify the ability of the trunk muscles to control lumbopelvic posture.[176] The test examines the ability of the trunk muscles to hold the lumbopelvic region in a steady position during progressive levels of leg loading, and were based on those reported by Sahrmann.[294,295] A key element of these tests is the precontraction of the deep muscles via a drawing in of the abdominal wall in preparation for the load and maintaining a neutral lumbar spine position (i.e. no posterior pelvic tilt). The measurement is conducted with the subject in the supine crook lying position, as this permits monitoring of the stable or unstable lumbopelvic position with the applied leg load without extraneous movement variables arising from body sway and balance.

The pressure biofeedback is an essential element of the test for it is placed under the lumbar spine to detect movement of the lumbo-pelvic region (see Appendix). The pressure biofeedback assesses where movement away from neutral occurs. For example, posterior pelvic tilt is reflected by an increasing pressure from the baseline pressure. Arching or extension of the lumbar spine and/or anterior pelvic tilt is reflected in a decrease in pressure from baseline. When the leg-load test emphasizes a rotatory bias, the bag is positioned longitudinally just lateral to the lumbar spine; if leg-loading is directed more in the sagittal plane, the bag is placed across the lumbar spine, with its base at the S2 level.[174,176,280,358] Inflation of the bag to a pressure of 40 mmHg after the patient has been positioned in supine crook lying, has been found clinically to be appropriate to fill the space between the irregularly shaped surface of the lumbar spine and the firm testing surface, but not to predisplace the lumbar spine from its natural resting position.

In addition to the use of a pressure bio-feedback unit to monitor and give immediate feedback of any loss of lumbopelvic position during the test, the shape of the abdominal wall is observed. An important feature of the test of lumbopelvic control is that the abdominal drawing-in action is performed first, prior to adding leg loading, and must be held (keeping the abdomen flat) throughout the entire test. This is a reflection of the ability of the transversus abdominis to hold in the abdominal contents as well as support and secure the lumbopelvic region.

The tests of lumbopelvic control can be graded from very low-load tests of short lever leg loading (Fig. 8.10) to higher load tests involving monitoring of lumbopelvic control through a leg-extension task. The patient is asked to watch the reading on the pressure gauge from the outset of the test. The pressure in the unit will rise slightly when the patient precontracts the deep muscles with an abdominal drawing-in action. The patient is asked to maintain this pressure reading during the test procedure, reflecting a steady position of the lumbopelvic region, and to keep the abdomen flat. It should be noted that the patient is not instructed to perform a backward tilt of the

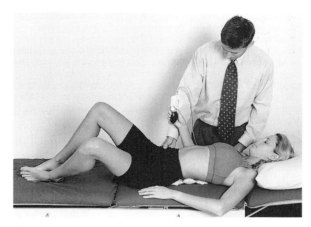

**Figure 8.10**   Low rotatory loads are used to test the control of lumbopelvic posture. Loads are imparted by requesting the patient to abduct and externally rotate one hip while the leg remains supported on the testing surface.

pelvis, which is commonly associated with leg-loading exercises, but rather to control the neutral position of the lumbopelvic region throughout the test. Leg load is added incrementally (Fig. 8.11). When the leg load exceeds the muscle capacity, the pressure registered on the gauge changes (either up or down, depending on the side of the spine on which the load has been placed or, if placed across the lower back, depending on whether the patient has moved into anterior or posterior pelvic tilt). Simultaneously, it will be observed that the patient can no longer keep the abdomen drawn in, and the abdominal wall bulges. When the leg load is at a manageable level, the transversus abdominis and lumbar multifidus do not contract in isolation during the tests, but all the abdominal muscles are activated together (to varying degrees) to control the stability of the lumbopelvic region. The low-load tests provide a more sensitive assessment of trunk muscle supporting capacity, as they better target the regional muscles. In higher load tests, muscles of adjacent and more remote areas are often recruited in response to the higher loads. These latter tests are more applicable in the later stages of a rehabilitation programme of a patient whose occupation or recreational activity requires strength in general trunk muscle support for high-load functional activities.

Some research has been undertaken to evaluate this clinical test. Wohlfahrt et al[358] used the leg-loading test in the supine lying position to test its relationship to the abdominal curl-up exercise. The research was conducted on army personnel who regularly perform high repetitions of curl-ups for their fitness assessment. The results revealed that those personnel who normally performed the repetitive curl-ups at a high rate scored significantly lower on the level of leg loading than did those who normally repeated the curl-up exercises at a slower rate. This indicated that high levels of lumbopelvic stabilization were not concomitant with the fast curl-up exercise. The results also suggested that a separate test was required to gain insight into the muscle supporting capacity of the lumbopelvic region, which was not reflected in the performance of a set number of curl-ups.

In another study, we investigated the control of lumbopelvic posture where the leg-loading tests were undertaken under two conditions: automatic control of lumbopelvic position under load, and control of the lumbopelvic position when subjects precontracted their deep trunk muscles by means of an abdominal drawing-in action.[176] A pressure sensor was used to monitor movement of the lumbopelvic region and the activity in the anterolateral abdominal wall was monitored using surface EMG. In the first instance, an index of the automatic ability of the trunk muscles to stabilize the trunk was obtained by noting the change from resting level pressure on assumption of a short lever unilateral leg load with the only pre-test instruction being to keep the trunk and pressure steady. The magnitude of change in pressure gave an index of general trunk muscle control. Ideally, there should be minimal change in pressure, indicating little lumbopelvic movement and a good ability of the trunk muscles to support the spine. The results between subjects were variable, with some showing little displacement while others demonstrated quite marked displacement, as evidenced by the pressure change. The test was repeated, but this time subjects were asked to precontract the deep trunk muscles by means of an abdominal drawing-in

(a)

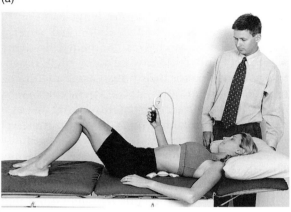

**Figure 8.11** The progression of leg load in tests of control of lumbopelvic posture. (a) Preparation for the test. The requirements of the test to keep the pressure as steady as possible and the importance of maintaining the deep muscle corset action during the test are explained to the patient. The patient is positioned in supine crook lying, with the legs together, or the legs abducted to emphasize rotatory control. The pressure sensor is positioned longitudinally on the side of the spine and inflated to 40 mmHg. The patient watches the pressure dial and draws in the abdominal wall. The pressure will increase slightly. The patient is instructed to keep the pressure level steady throughout the test. (b) Level 1: single leg slide, contralateral leg support. (Left) Leg slide with heel support to full extension and return. (Right) Unsupported leg slide: the heel is held approximately 5 cm from the exercise surface. (c) Level 2: Single leg slide, contralateral leg unsupported. (Left) Leg slide with heel support to full extension and return. (Right) Unsupported leg slide: the heel is held approximately 5 cm from exercise surface.

(b)

(c)

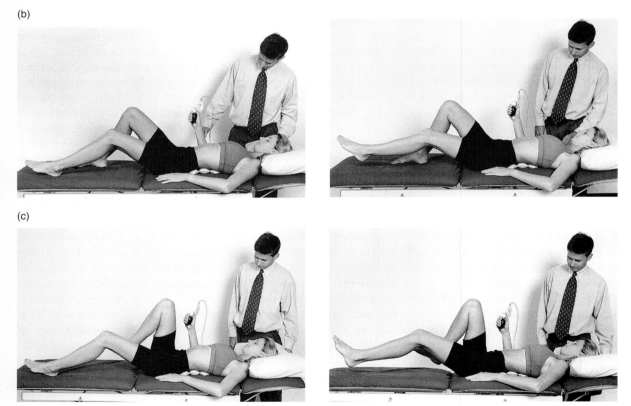

action. The difference in magnitude between the pressure changes under the two test conditions provided an estimate of the effect of presetting the abdominal muscles prior to leg loading. Subjects who were deemed to have poor control of their lumbopelvic region (large changes in pressure in the first automatic test) significantly improved their performance with the pre-contraction required in the second test. This suggested that the automatic function of the muscles involved in drawing in the abdominal wall were not used to their full capacity. Conversely, subjects who showed small pressure changes in the automatic test showed virtually no change with the conscious preactivation of their deep muscles in the second test, suggesting that these muscles were functioning adequately and automatically. These results also support the suggestion that the deep muscles play some part in providing rotatory control of the lumbo-pelvic region (see Ch. 4).

These tests of lumbopelvic postural control permit some quantification in the clinical setting of the supporting capacity of muscles, which has not been possible previously, and can be used to guide treatment decisions to ensure safe progression of exercise. In addition, tests of the control of lumbopelvic position can be used to assess the effectiveness of exercise that focuses on the interaction of the local and global muscle systems under load (see Ch. 10).

## DEVELOPMENT OF THE THREE-TIER SYSTEM

The clinical measures have been developed over the past several years from research done in our laboratory as well as through clinical practice. Such a level of assessment has been directed for use by clinicians only as, although some features can be quantified, the conduct and interpretation of the tests are enhanced by skilled observation of the body contours, palpation of deep muscle action and analysis of the type of breathing patterns, skills that are familiar to physical therapists. These tests have their limitations, for a number of reasons. On the one hand, there is a need for 'user-friendly' screening tests that require minimal equipment and minimal operator skill for widespread use on large population groups in work or sports screening or in gymnasiums (see screening tests in Fig. 8.1). At the highest level, detailed assessments of motor-control deficits are required in which the use of observation and palpation are minimized, being replaced by more objective measurements. Such tests are needed for outcome measures for research purposes and for a level of diagnosis

requiring definitive evidence and quantification of the problem. We have called these tests diagnostic assessments (see Fig. 8.1).

### Diagnostic assessments

At present, the most direct diagnostic method of measuring motor-control deficits in the transversus abdominis and the final output of segmental levels of the multifidus is assessment by EMG using fine-wire electrodes placed within the target muscles. This method measures how the nervous system controls the contractions of the deep muscles, through the use of a reaction task involving arm or leg movements in the standing position. The temporal patterns of the deep muscles give an objective means of assessing whether motor-control deficits are present in the deep muscles in back pain patients. This method is based on the one described by Hodges & Richardson.[146,147] While this is an invasive assessment, it has the advantage of measuring the automatic function of the muscles during the specific task, and does not summon the variable of patient volition.

A second diagnostic method, which has the advantage of being non-invasive, has been developed from the volitional clinical measures. It involves assessing the level and type of muscle action during the motor skills of drawing in the abdominal wall, isometrically contracting the segmental lumbar multifidus and the leg-loading tests. By combining the outputs from various types of measurement apparatus, more objective information is gained about the motor-control problems in the low back pain patient. The measurement employs the simultaneous use of real-time ultrasound imaging, collection of analogue data from a pressure biofeedback unit connected to a pressure transducer and surface EMG (Fig. 8.12).

In the motor skill of drawing in the abdominal wall, the interaction of the abdominal muscle layers and the control of the action of the transversus abdominis to contract into its shortened range are assessed using ultrasound imaging and pressure changes. Simultaneously, the level of any unwanted activity in the global muscles

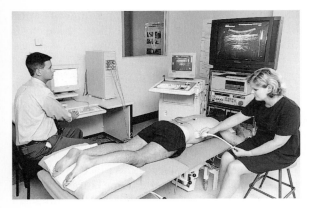

**Figure 8.12** Non-invasive measurement of deep muscle activation using ultrasound imaging, pressure and surface EMG. (Patent pending, The University of Queensland.)

during the test manoeuvre is documented using surface EMG. The three measures serve to define the problem and to provide definitive treatment strategies to address the particular problem of the individual patient. The combination of real-time ultrasound imaging and surface EMG is used to assess the patient's ability to activate the segmental level of the lumbar multifidus in a slow, controlled, low level contraction. Ultrasound imaging provides the opportunity to distinguish noninvasively deep from superficial fibre activity within the multifidus muscle.

While quantifiable diagnostic measures have been developed, before they can be adopted for general use in diagnosis of motor control problems in low back pain patients, the results of the assessments need to be evaluated with the rigour of scientific investigation in order to assess their validity and ability to detect differences between people with and without low back pain. The development of these detailed and more objective measures seems particularly relevant to those problematic patients having recurrent or chronic low back pain and who do not respond readily to conservative treatment. These detailed assessments appear to have the capacity to define the deep muscle capacity objectively, and also accurately to detect the nature and extent of any substitution strategies. Provision of such data can guide and direct

therapeutic exercise treatments more effectively and efficiently.

## FUTURE DIRECTIONS

The clinical outcome of evidence-based practices depend on having sensitive and specific measures of motor-control problems in back pain patients. The invasive tests provide the main solution to this problem of measurement. However, assessments involving needle insertion, while useful for laboratory research, are not likely to appeal to the general back pain population at this time. The non-invasive assessments involve patient volition and, thereby, also have limitations. Nevertheless, due to the significance of the findings of deficits in the local muscle system of low back pain patients, it is essential that suitable outcome measures be determined. For this reason the various levels of assessment described in this chapter are under continual development and are being subjected to extensive scrutiny in order to establish their reliability and validity to allow their future use in clinical research directed towards determining optimal treatments for back pain patients as well as investigations on the most effective methods of back pain prevention.

## APPENDIX: DEVELOPMENT OF PRESSURE BIOFEEDBACK

During the development of the initial clinical tests of stabilization function, it was necessary to develop a device that could monitor the position (i.e. stable or unstable) of the lumbopelvic region during leg-loading tests performed with the patient in the supine position. A direct measure of the complex three-dimensional motion of the lumbopelvic region is not easy, and thus an indirect method was developed for clinical testing (Stabilizer, Chattanooga South Pacific). The pressure biofeedback unit[283] consists of an inelastic, three-section air-filled bag, which is inflated to fill the space between the target body area and a firm surface, and a pressure dial for monitoring the pressure in the bag for feedback

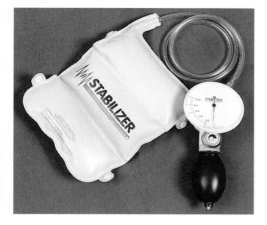

**Figure 8.13** The pressure biofeedback unit consists of a three-section, inelastic inflatable pad with a pressure pump and dial.

on position (Fig. 8.13). The bag is inflated to an appropriate level for the purpose and the pressure recorded. Quite simply, movement of the body part off the bag results in a decrease in pressure, while movement of the body part onto the bag results in an increase in pressure.

The device has come into general use for stabilization exercises for all parts of the body. Its use in assessing the abdominal drawing-in action has, however, become its most important use in relation to the treatment of problems of the local muscle system in low back pain patients. A method was needed to gain some quantification of the abdominal drawing-in action in the clinic, and the pressure biofeedback unit was found to meet this need. As the transversus abdominis produces narrowing of the abdominal wall, measurement of the amount of movement of the abdomen that can be produced provides a method of identifying a patient's ability to perform the contraction. To under-

stand this, it is necessary to consider the orientation of the abdominal muscles.

The majority of the muscle fibres of the rectus abdominis, obliquus externus abdominis and obliquus internus abdominis run either vertically or obliquely from the pelvis to the rib cage. When these muscles contract they can flatten the abdominal wall, but do not narrow the waist beyond this. In contrast, the fibres of the transversus abdominis are horizontal and can therefore produce a concavity of the abdominal wall without movement of the spine. Thus when the transversus abdominis contracts in isolation, concavity of the abdominal wall results, whereas substitution by the other abdominal muscles simply flattens the abdomen. Measurement of the elevation of the abdominal wall from the supporting surface, with the patient in the prone position, allows identification of both how well the transversus abdominis can be contracted and whether this action can be performed in isolation. The motion is assessed using the pressure biofeedback unit.

The principle underlying the use of the pressure biofeedback unit in this test is that, when the unit is placed under the abdomen, it initially conforms to the patient's shape. As the patient draws in the stomach off the pad, the pressure in the pad is reduced. The pressure reduction is proportional to the degree to which the patient can elevate the abdominal wall. The specific construction of this device has considerable advantages. First, since the material is inelastic it can accurately reflect abdominal wall motion without distortion. This is assisted by the partitioning of the device into three sections, which assists with the distribution of the air within the pad. When the device is positioned appropriately, the shape of the pad permits an evaluation to be made of the movement of the abdomen.

# 9

# Analysis and treatment of motor-control problems in the local muscles of the lumbopelvic region

There are possibly many ways of approaching the treatment of motor-control problems in back pain patients. The approach described here is not based on theoretical concepts alone, but has evolved from working with back pain patients in the clinical and the laboratory situation. The emergence of ultrasound imaging and electromyography (EMG) have permitted real-time viewing and recording of the activity of all muscle layers. This has increased our ability to analyse the patterns of muscle usage in the standard clinical tests, which also enables treatment strategies to be applied more precisely and efficiently. As described previously, treatment may consist of three stages: formal motor skill training of the deep muscles; incorporation of the skill into light functional tasks; and progression to heavy functional tasks. This chapter describes the formal motor skill training. The integration of the deep muscle co-contraction pattern into dynamic function is described in Chapter 10.

## FORMAL SKILL TRAINING

Clinical examination reveals that low back pain patients do not have the motor skill of performing an isometric continuous co-contraction of the transversus abdominis and the lumbar multifidus independently of the action of the global muscles. The elements for relearning a motor skill and for progressing the treatment to the integration stage were described in Chapter 7 (see Fig. 7.4).

There is a process of clinical problem-solving

that is undertaken in preparation for prescribing the exercise and facilitation strategies, a process that must continue throughout the whole rehabilitation period. The individual nature and extent of the global muscle overactivity, detected as unwanted global muscle activity during attempts to perform the skill, directs the selection of the most expedient treatment for the individual patient.

The clinical presentation of the low back pain patient, in terms of muscle dysfunction, seems to fall into two basic categories. One group presents with lack of control in muscles of the local system. Their global muscles are either normal or exhibit a lack of strength and endurance. The second group also presents with lack of control in muscles of the local system but, in contrast, their global muscles do not appear to have primary problems in strength or endurance (Fig. 9.1). In fact, various muscles of the global system appear to be overactive. This is evidenced by a marked degree of unwanted activity during attempts to perform deep muscle co-contraction. Clinical practice suggests that patients in the second group offer the greater

challenge to the therapeutic skills of the practitioner, as these patients appear to have greater problems. The relationship between trunk muscle overactivity, local motor control problems and the degree of passive insufficiency in the spinal osseoligamentous system is an important area of future research.

In approaching treatment, the clinician must answer two basic questions:

- Does the patient present with unwanted global muscle activity?
- If so, which muscles are problematic?

These questions need to be answered in order to institute best-practice therapeutic exercise. For patients without unwanted overactivity in the global muscles, the clinician can simply choose the best ways of activating the local muscle system. However, in patients with unwanted global muscle overactivity, the clinician must choose strategies that simultaneously reduce the unwanted global muscle activity while activating the co-contraction in the local muscles for spinal segmental support. To this end, the clinician must undertake an additional process to analyse the nature and extent of the unwanted global muscle activity. Elements of this process for recognition of individual presentations is described separately and in some detail in this text. Once the clinician becomes skilled, the process is not time consuming, as the analysis and treatment proceed together.

## Signs of unwanted global muscle activation

Careful analytical observation of the trunk manoeuvres can give an indication of any marked substitution by the global muscles, and these observations can be made either during the tests or on other occasions of convenience where the abdominal wall can be viewed in its entirety. The most commonly overactive global muscle identified to date which substitutes for the transversus abdominis and lumbar multifidus is the obliquus externus abdominis. The obliquus internus abdominis, rectus abdominis and thoracic portions of the erector spinae may

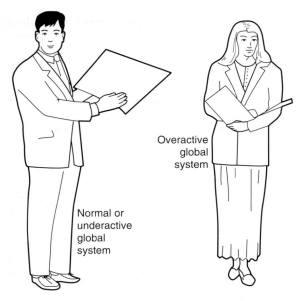

Overactive global system

Normal or underactive global system

**Figure 9.1** The two general categories of muscle dysfunction in low back pain patients.

also present problems. The following discussion is not exhaustive and the clinician should be aware that other unique strategies may present in an individual patient and should be corrected. Substitution can be detected by observing aberrant trunk movements and contours, by palpation and by EMG.

### Spinal movement

*Note: The specific co-contraction of the transversus abdominis and deep portions of the lumbar multifidus does not produce spinal movement.*

Contraction of the obliquus externus abdominis and rectus abdominis may produce backward pelvic tilting and flexion of the trunk. In the prone position test, any observed slight flexion of the thoracolumbar and lumbopelvic area could be caused by the action of these muscles instead of the transversus abdominis. The movement at the thoracolumbar junction is often very subtle, and palpating for movement is a useful adjunct to observation. In addition, a quite rapid reduction in pressure (as indicated by the pressure biofeedback unit; see Appendix, Ch. 8) during the test could signal flexion of the spine and indicate a dominance in these muscles.

A slight backward pelvic tilting action can be substituted for the correct swelling-out action during the isometric test of the segmental lumbar multifidus. This is the most common substitution seen clinically. The patient attempts to push too hard posteriorly, and flexes the lumbar spine. Another substitution strategy involves a slight anterior pelvic tilt at the lumbosacral junction. This occurs when the patient predominantly uses the more superficial multifidus fibres in the contraction, causing the spine to extend. Patients often report this type of contraction to be painful. Maximal contraction of all the multifidus fascicles in concert with the lumbar erector spinae muscles can generate an anterior shearing force at the lumbosacral junction.[39] Even though the contraction is not maximal in the test attempt, this substitution must be detected. If the patient performs the lumbar multifidus contraction incorrectly, too vigorously and without co-activation of the

transversus abdominis, *there is a potential to aggravate the patient's pain.*

### The rib cage

Further indications of substitution strategies can be gained by observing the movement of the rib cage during the abdominal drawing-in action with the patient in a standing or supine crook lying position. The muscle fibres of the obliquus externus abdominis originate from the external surface of the lower ribs, unlike those of the transversus abdominis, which originate from the internal surface. Contraction of the anteromedial fibres of the obliquus externus abdominis produces a downward and inward movement of the rib cage, which is observed as a subtle depression in its ventral aspect.

### The abdominal wall

Observation of the entire abdominal wall during the contraction can also give a good indication of any predominance of the obliquus externus abdominis. When teaching the abdominal drawing-in action in the four-point kneeling position, in the prone test or in other positions such as supine crook lying or standing, dominant activity in the obliquus externus abdominis can be observed when movement of the abdominal wall is initiated or predominates in the upper quadrants rather than the lower quadrants below the navel. The formation of a transverse fold in the upper abdomen is another indication of an overactive obliquus externus abdominis, and contraction of the muscle fibres at their origin on the rib cage may be observed (Fig. 9.2). Another sign that the obliquus externus abdominis may be overactive is an increase in the lateral diameter of the abdominal wall commensurate with a subtle abdominal bracing manoeuvre, and this can be identified by palpation of the lateral abdominal wall bilaterally during the performance of the contraction. In addition, on palpation, tightness in longitudinally directed fibres in the anterolateral abdomen is a common sign of obliquus externus abdominis substitution. It can also be useful to

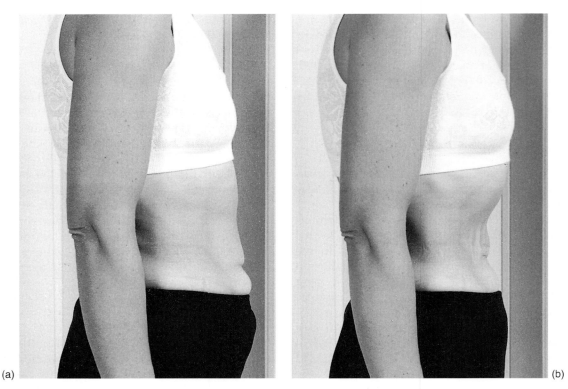

(a)                                                                                          (b)

**Figure 9.2**    (a) Abdomen relaxed. (b) Dominant contraction of the obliquus externus abdominis, indicated by a transverse fold or skin crease just superior to the umbilicus.

palpate over the muscle fibres of the rectus abdominis anteriorly during the performance of the contraction in order to assess any contribution of this muscle to the drawing-in action, which may be subtle.

### Breathing pattern

We have observed clinically that the breathing pattern can be altered in chronic low back pain patients. The oblique abdominals are sometimes active during both inspiration and expiration. These muscles should normally be relaxed during the breathing cycle, except during forced expiration.[83,145] As a clinical observation, low back pain patients find it difficult to activate the transversus abdominis in isolation if the oblique abdominal muscles are active during the breathing cycle. Furthermore, we have also observed that some low back pain patients are

able to draw in their abdominal wall successfully, but are then unable to maintain the contraction once they try to resume breathing. It therefore seems important to try to establish a diaphragmatic pattern of breathing and to decrease activity in the oblique abdominal muscles before attempting to train the patient in isolated contraction of the transversus abdominis. An altered breathing pattern seems to be an indicator of patients who will be more difficult to facilitate and train.

### Unwanted activity in the back extensors

An increase in activity of the thoracic portions of the erector spinae, observed in prone lying or standing, in either the abdominal drawing-in test or in the test of isometric segmental lumbar multifidus contraction, can be another sign of muscle substitution. The presence of this contraction with the obliquus externus abdominis and rectus abdominis, or this contraction instead of that of the lumbar multifidus, suggests that the patient requires or uses this global muscle pattern to maintain the neutral position of the spine, instead of the more appropriate use of the deep muscle system.

### Summary

In summary, recognition of physical signs of unwanted global muscle activity signals to the clinician which postures, movements and instructions to avoid during the facilitation and training of the deep muscle activation. (See Box 9.1.)

## REHABILITATION OF THE MOTOR SKILL

For normal function, the transversus abdominis and the deep fibres of the lumbar multifidus must be modulated continuously to control the lumbar spinal segments independently of the contractions of the global muscles, which produce the trunk and pelvic movements. The first step is to give formal exercises to train the patient to contract the deep muscles cognitively, and to ensure that the transversus abdominis and lumbar multifidus can contract independently of the global muscles. To allow the patient to learn the correct deep muscle activation skill as efficiently as possible, the most suitable instructions, body positions and techniques of facilitation are chosen for the individual patient.

## Instructions and teaching cues

The patient must be provided with a clear explanation of the nature of muscle activity required for joint support, the need for particular muscles to be performing this task and, therefore, the precision required in training. Since the level of contraction required is minor in comparison to the conventional images of exercise for strength training or cardiovascular fitness, it is necessary continually to impress on the patient concepts of motor control and skill training. An explanation of the need to change the way the brain is using the muscle rather than increasing the muscle strength is helpful. A description of the effort required in the muscle to support the joints (e.g. 10–15% of maximum effort) helps to convey the aims of precision and control of muscle activity and the need for endurance.

As a component of the initial teaching phase prior to testing, the clinician will have already taken time to explain and demonstrate the contraction to the patient. The use of diagrams and models is effective at this stage. A demonstration by the clinician of the correct contraction of the transversus abdominis and lumbar multifidus with the patient observing or palpating the correct action is also very useful. The patient then perceives from the outset the subtlety and precise nature of the contractions involved. The sequence used in the testing procedure is still followed in training; i.e. the patient takes in a relaxed breath, breathes out gently, ceases breathing while he or she attempts to activate the deep muscles, and then resumes a relaxed

---

**Box 9.1**   Physical signs of unwanted global muscle activity

Aberrant movement
- Posterior pelvic tilt
- Flexion of the thoracolumbar junction
- Rib cage depression

Contours of the abdominal wall
- No movement of the lower abdomen
- Increased lateral diameter of the abdominal wall
- Visible contraction of the obliquus externus abdominis muscle fibres at their origin
- Patient unable voluntarily to relax the abdominal wall

Aberrant breathing patterns
- Inappropriate activation of the obliquus externus abdominis and obliquus internus abdominis during the breathing cycle
- Patient unable to perform diaphragmatic breathing pattern

Unwanted activity of the back extensors
- Co-activation of the thoracic portions of the erector spinae

Methods of detection
- Observation
- Palpation
- EMG

> **Box 9.2** Examples of instructions
>
> Transversus abdominis
> - Slowly draw in your lower abdomen away from the elastic of your pants.
> - Slowly draw in your lower abdomen to support the weight of the abdominal contents [prone].
> - Slowly draw your navel up and in towards your backbone.
> - Slowly pull in your abdominal contents to gently flatten your stomach below your navel [standing].
>
> Lumbar multifidus
> - Gently swell out or contract your muscle against my fingers.

breathing pattern while holding the contraction. It is a matter of trial and error to find the instruction that correctly cues the patient. Some example instructions are given in Box 9.2.

Tactile cues assist in teaching the isometric contraction of the lumbar multifidus at the segmental level. This can be provided by the clinician or patient (Fig. 9.3). Care should be taken to gently but firmly sink the thumb and/or fingers deeply into the muscle bellies adjacent to the spinous process in order to facilitate the contraction. Accurate feedback on correct performance can be gained by feeling a deep and slowly generated tension developing under the fingers as the muscle swells out in response to the resistance. Feeling a rapid or superficial contraction may indicate either contraction of the longer

superficial fibres of the multifidus or tension in the tendinous portion of the thoracic erector spinae which span the lumbar area.

Tactile cues for teaching the contraction of transversus abdominis are very useful, but are more indirect as the muscle is deep and is overlaid by the obliquus internus abdominis and externus. The ideal position for tactile cues is anterior and inferior to the anterior superior iliac spines and lateral to the rectus abdominis. The thumbs or middle three fingers are used to sink gently but deeply into the abdominal wall (Fig. 9.4). Either the clinician or the patient can use the technique. This position cues the patient to the lower abdomen, and recent evidence suggests that the lower portion of the transversus abdominis may be the part most essential for spinal stabilization.[144] With a correct contraction of the transversus abdominis, the clinician feels a slowly developing deep tension in the abdominal wall (Fig 9.5). With an incorrect action, the clinician may find one of three conditions on palpation. There may be no activity. A dominance or substitution by the oblique abdominals may be palpated via a rapid development of tension in the abdominal wall, a superficial muscle contraction, or the palpating fingers are pushed out of the abdominal wall by a bracing action including all the lateral abdominals (Fig 9.5c). Another anomaly is palpation of an abnormal left/right asymmetry in the contraction of transversus abdominis.

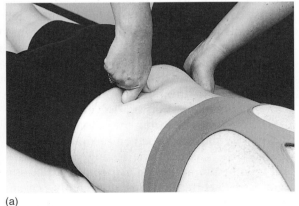

(a)

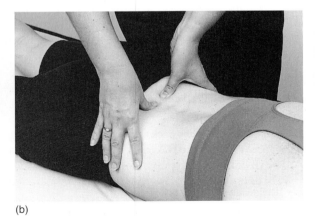

(b)

**Figure 9.3** Two hand positions for tactile facilitation of the segmental lumbar multifidus.

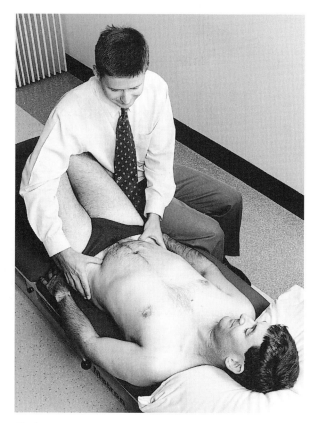

**Figure 9.4**  The hand position for palpation during transversus abdominis activation.

The action of the transversus abdominis can be also be mimicked by sucking in the abdominal wall and reducing the intrathoracic pressure without contracting the transversus abdominis. When a deep breath is taken by increasing the lateral diameter of the rib cage or by increasing the upper chest volume through the use of the accessory respiratory muscles (e.g. the scalenes and sternocleidomastoid), the volume of the thorax is increased. This has the potential to elevate the diaphragm, in addition to producing inward movement of air. The consequence of this upward diaphragm movement is inward movement of the abdominal wall, giving the appearance of contraction of transversus abdominis (Fig 9.6). Since the abdominal wall movement is performed passively, no palpable contraction or tightening of any muscle of the abdominal wall will be perceived.

## Body position

Due to the orientation and mechanics of the muscle fibres of the transversus abdominis and, in particular, the deep fibres of the mutifidus, the actions of these muscles are independent of spinal posture and their length–tension relationship is not affected by spinal position.[219] This means that, with back pain patients, any spinal or lumbopelvic posture can be adopted to teach and train the muscle contractions in the first instance. Various options are available, including side lying, supine crook lying, standing, sitting, supported high sitting, four-point kneeling, and standing or sitting leaning forwards while weight bearing through the arms. The choice of position is by trial and error. It is based on controlling factors which could otherwise be detrimental to performance (e.g. unwanted global muscle activity) or, conversely, helpful to the patient to achieve the local muscle action. Body positioning alters the load on the spinal structures. The patient should be pain-free in the position chosen, as pain during the muscle activation strategy may invoke muscle inhibition. Non-weight-bearing positions also take load off the global muscles, which is very desirable if they are overactive and substituting for the action of the deep target muscles. The effects of gravity combined with the weight of the abdominal contents, e.g. in side lying, might be useful in providing a stretch stimulus to transversus abdominis activation. The position chosen must also help promote good and relaxed breathing patterns; the reasons for this will become evident in subsequent sections. The side lying or three-quarters prone position may also be useful for the facilitation of the lumbar multifidus.

## Additional methods of facilitation

When a patient is unable to perform an isolated contraction of the transversus abdominis or segmental lumbar multifidus with a simple instruction of the required action, or if the patient is

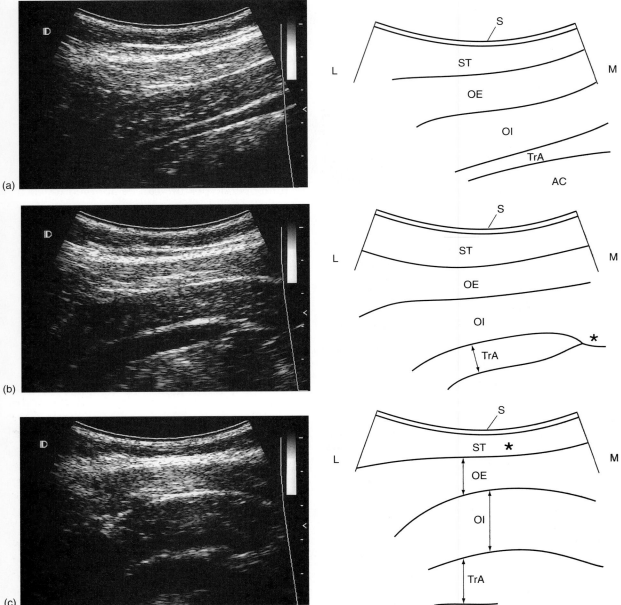

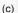

**Figure 9.5** An inside view of the palpatory cues. Ultrasound images of the abdominal wall in transverse section (transducer placed anterolaterally). (a) Relaxed abdominal wall. Note the curved skin (S) line due to the convex shape of the transducer. (b) Abdominal wall following performance of the correct drawing-in action (palpation: deep tension in the abdominal wall). On contraction of the transversus abdominis (TrA), the muscle increases in depth ($\updownarrow$) and tensions the fascia, which attaches to rectus abdominis (*). There is little change in the superficial muscles (obliquus externus abdominis (OE) and obliquus internus abdominis (OI). On palpation, deep tension is felt in the abdominal wall as the TrA pulls the lower abdomen in. (c) Abdominal wall following incorrect performance of drawing-in action (palpation: pushing out action of the abdominal wall). Note the increased depth of the OE, OI and TrA ($\leftrightarrow$) as the isolated activation of the TrA is lost. The distance from the superior border of the OE to the skin is decreased as the patient pushes out (*). On palpation, the fingers are pushed outwards. AC, abdominal contents; L, lateral; M, medial; ST, subcutaneous tissue.

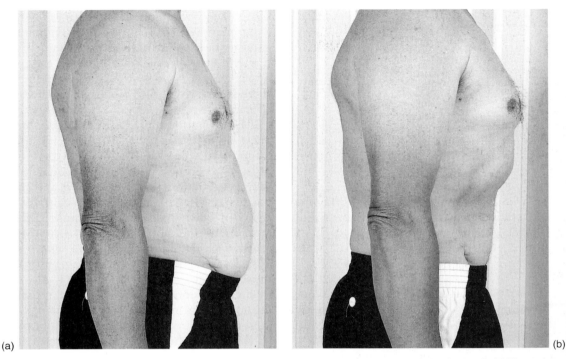

(a)                                                                          (b)

**Figure 9.6**    A substitution strategy for the abdominal drawing-in action. (a) A relaxed abdominal wall. (b) The action of the transversus abdominis is mimicked by sucking in the abdominal wall.

having difficulty controlling a substitution strategy, the next step is to facilitate this contraction. The key to facilitation of transversus abdominis and lumbar multifidus contraction is careful teaching of the actions, with specific attention to the correction of compensations. If a substitution is allowed to persist, then the isolation of transversus abdominis or lumbar multifidus has not been achieved, and training of the optimal strategy for trunk control will not occur at the same rate or with the same success. There are several techniques that can be used to assist with this isolation and the correction of substitutions. These techniques are based on principles of motor control and neuromuscular physiology, and represent the culmination of various research projects and clinical expertise. The principle of these techniques is essentially to allow the patient to achieve the best possible contraction in the early stages. As soon as possible, the clinician should aim to have the patient gain cognitive control of the transversus abdominis and lumbar multifidus

without needing to rely on any facilitation technique. Thus, facilitation provides an intermediate but essential step in the path to achieving cognitive control. As with any manual therapy technique, a high level of skill and precision is required by the clinician to master these facilitation techniques, and the clinician must be willing to practise the techniques in order to gain proficiency in their use.

The patient needs to gain a perception of the contraction prior to performing precise repetitions of the action. In the beginning, most patients cannot perceive or appreciate the deep muscle contraction and require facilitation. While the outcome is to facilitate the co-activation of the transversus abdominis and lumbar multifidus, strategies often focus the patient's attention to particular elements of the motor skill for easier learning. There are several facilitation techniques that have been demonstrated to be useful clinically in treating back pain patients. The clinician must appreciate that treatment needs to be tailored to

---

**Box 9.3** Points of technique

- The clinician must master the skill of facilitation.
- The clinician should persist for the independent co-contraction of the transversus abdominis and lumbar multidfidus.
- The patient should aim for cognitive control without relying on facilitation techniques.
- The treatment should be tailored to the individual patient.

---

the individual patient in order to find the strategy (or strategies) to which the patient best responds. (See Box 9.3.)

*Contraction of stability synergists*

It appears that four key muscle groups may work in synergy: the transversus abdominis, lumbar multifidus, the pelvic floor and diaphragm (see Chs 4 and 7). An explanation to patients of the cylinder-like effect that these muscles have in their supporting role in the lumbopelvic region helps them to understand the use and interplay of the activation of these muscles in facilitatory strategies (see Fig. 7.4, Ch. 7). In fact, any one of the four muscles can be used to help facilitate another.

**Transversus abdominis and lumbar multifidus.** The co-activation of the transversus abdominis and the lumbar multifidus can be utilized quite successfully in facilitation. If the patient cognitively achieves the contraction of either the transversus abdominis or the lumbar multifidus more readily, then the successful muscle contraction can be used to facilitate the other one. Very simply, if the patient cannot consciously activate the transversus abdominis, then the clinician tries to achieve activation through facilitation of the lumbar multifidus or, conversely, focuses on the activation of transversus abdominis to facilitate lumbar multifidus. Logically, the contraction of the primary muscle must be performed well to achieve the desired result. For example, a phasic and poorly executed multifidus contraction may result in co-activation of the oblique abdominal muscles rather than the

transversus abdominis. The clinician may need to experiment with patient position to find the ideal combination for the individual patient.

**Pelvic floor.** Use of contraction of the muscles of the pelvic floor is one of the most effective methods of achieving isolation of the contraction of the transversus abdominis. In order for the transversus abdominis to contribute to stabilization of the spine, it is essential for the contraction of the diaphragm and pelvic floor muscles to occur concurrently in order to maintain the abdominal contents within the abdominal cavity. Preliminary studies (see Ch. 4) have revealed that, when a limb is moved, the contraction of the pubococcygeus occurs concurrently with that of the transversus abdominis. It appears that a link may exist between these two muscles. Several researchers have also noted that contraction of the abdominal muscles, in particular the transversus abdominis, is associated with contraction of the pelvic floor muscles in retraining the pelvic floor muscles for the management of urinary stress incontinence.[297] Other clinical evidence is emerging of a relationship between transversus abdominis and the pelvic floor. This has arisen from claims from patients that their stress incontinence problem has reduced following a course of exercises for the transversus abdominis and, conversely, people managed for stress incontinence reporting a reduced incidence of low back pain. The use of contraction of the pelvic floor muscles to facilitate contraction of the transversus abdominis is particularly useful in patients who are having difficulty understanding the movement that is required to contract the transversus abdominis. It is also a primary technique for those who cannot relax their obliquus externus abdominis in the abdominal drawing-in task.

Contraction of the pelvic floor can be utilized in a number of ways. It can be used either in isolation without the addition of a cognitive transversus abdominis contraction, or by combining the pelvic floor contraction with a cognitive contraction of the transversus abdominis or other facilitation techniques. With the implementation of this facilitation strategy it is important first to teach an effective contraction of the pelvic floor muscles. Many methods are available to do this, although the principles of slow, gentle and low effort of contraction should be employed. A clear description of the anatomy as a muscular sling between the tail bone and the front of the pelvis is essential to assist the patient to visualize the contraction. The reader is referred to Sapsford et al[297] for a more detailed description of methods of achieving contraction of the pelvic floor muscles. The clinician is advised to use whatever techniques they have within their competence and they deem necessary to achieve the correct contraction.

Supine crook lying or side lying seem to be the better positions for initial teaching of the pelvic floor contraction, although the strategy can certainly be used in standing or sitting. The clinician and/or patient gently, but deeply, palpates the lower quadrant of the abdomen. The sequence used is identical to that described before, where the patient takes in a relaxed breath, breathes out gently and then draws the pelvic floor up slowly and gently. The clinician feels for the deep tension developing in the abdominal wall as the transversus abdominis co-activates with the pelvic floor. A rapidly developing or superficial tension in the abdominal wall usually accompanies a fast or inadequate attempt at contraction of the pelvic floor, and signals substitution with the global muscles. The feedback provided to the patient by self-palpation of the abdominal wall can be quite potent towards their understanding of the synergistic muscle facilitation strategy.

With the aim of this stage of management being to train transversus abdominis activation in isolation from the other global abdominal muscles, activation via the pelvic floor alone is often sufficient in the early stages of rehabilitation. This is so when the obliquus externus abdominis is overactive and any attempt to extend the synergistic contraction into the abdomen results in this global muscle activity. As soon as possible, the patient is taught to consciously extend the contraction up into the lower abdomen and draw in the lower abdominal wall. Self-monitoring with palpation for the desired response in the abdominal wall is essential in

the learning process for cognitive control of the transversus abdominis.

Conscious interplay between initiation of a pelvic floor contraction followed by a gentle reinforcement of the transversus abdominis contraction and then back to focus on the pelvic floor can increase awareness of both muscles. If the patient has trouble achieving a pelvic floor contraction, other methods with which the clinician is familiar should be tried to assist with activation.

Pelvic floor contraction can also be used to teach and facilitate an isometric contraction of the segmental multifidus. It is particularly helpful when the patient has a poor awareness of the multifidus muscle, the lumbar segment as well as the desired muscle contraction. Facilitation can either be attempted in side or prone lying, or standing. It is usually attempted in a non-weight-bearing position first. While the clinician palpates the targeted vertebral level, the patient is asked to slowly draw up the pelvic floor. A slow and gentle deep tensioning of the multifidus muscle is the desired response. The contraction should slowly build in intensity and is therefore subtle to detect. If a quick contraction is palpated, it is likely that contraction of the superficial fibres has occurred. The subject should be encouraged to try again with less effort.

**Breathing patterns (diaphragm).** The role of transversus abdominis in the production of expiration can also be utilized to activate this muscle. Ideally, the only possible way to achieve isolation of the transversus abdominis during expiration is to increase the expiratory effort by hyperoxic hypercapnia (rebreathing $CO_2$),[83,347] or by the provision of an inspiratory load, which produces an involuntary increase in expiratory airflow.[83] Both produce an involuntary and selective increase in transversus abdominis activity during expiration to increase the expiratory airflow. However, in clinical practice it can be effective simply to instruct the patient to 'sigh' the air out during expiration and to draw up the abdomen as they do this. Since all the abdominal muscles are commonly activated with voluntary increases in expiratory flow,[83,145] careful assessment is needed to ensure the success of the technique in achieving an isolated contraction of the transversus abdominis. Future research may identify strategies that use the contraction of the diaphragm to facilitate directly transversus abdominis contraction.

Patients who overuse the obliquus externus abdominis will often increase this substitution with expiration. In such patients attention may need to be placed first on teaching relaxed diaphragmatic breathing. We have observed clinically that relaxed breathing can decrease global muscle activation, which in turn can allow activation of a transversus abdominis contraction (see p. 138).

### Verbal and visual feedback

It is vital to provide adequate verbal and visual feedback to the patient of their performance. In the motor control literature, this principle is known as the 'knowledge of performance' and 'knowledge of results'.[300] In patients who have had a cerebrovascular accident, it is imperative to provide this information because the patient has sustained an injury involving the kinesthetic sense. Studies have reported reduced kinesthetic acuity in people with low back pain,[266] which may compound learning problems. An added complication is that the performance of the abdominal drawing-in manoeuvre is not normally performed by an individual as a separate isolated task and is an unfamiliar action. Irrespective of whether or not the patient's kinesthetic sense has been affected by the back injury, provision of enhanced feedback appears be a critical factor required to achieve an isolated contraction of the transversus abdominis and segmental lumbar multifidus.

Direct visual feedback of the correct deep muscle contraction through the use of real-time ultrasound imaging is proving to be a very effective form of feedback in both teaching and learning of the action for the transversus abdominis and lumbar multifidus.[135,321] Imaging the muscles in real time gives a guarantee of the success, or otherwise, of a particular facilitation strategy. Opportunities exist for real-time ultrasound imaging techniques to be developed and

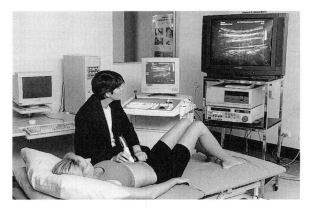

**Figure 9.7** The patient receives real-time feedback of the muscles of the anterolateral wall from the visual display unit.

used for each of the four deep muscles targeted in the rehabilitation of lumbopelvic control.

The contraction of the transversus abdominis and any substitution by the obliquus externus abdominis or obliquus internus abdominis can be observed by placing the transducer over the anterolateral abdominal wall to view the three muscle layers in transverse section (Fig. 9.7). The patient is orientated to the ultrasound image of the three muscle layers. The action to be observed with a correct transversus abdominis contraction is explained as the slow and controlled drawing in of this muscle in its corset-like action and appearance. This should occur with relative relaxation and little movement of the obliquus externus abdominis and obliquus internus abdominis. Simultaneous contraction of the three muscle layers as a single entity should not occur. When this does occur, the patient can realize his or her poor pattern of control and how the transversus abdominis has changed to work as a general abdominal muscle and not in its specific independent function (see Ch. 5). The effectiveness of various facilitation methods can be assessed until one which cues the patient successfully is observed. Meanwhile, the patient, in trying these methods to facilitate transversus abdominis activation, watches the real-time image of the muscle and palpates their lower abdominal wall to learn the correct muscle action. In addition their ability to hold the contraction can be observed and monitored, as can

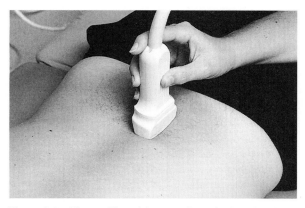

**Figure 9.8**  The position of the transducer for imaging the lumbar mutifidus in the parasagittal plane.

the time at which the muscle becomes fatigued and the isolated contraction is either lost or is joined by the contraction of obliquus externus abdominis or internus abdominis in substitution.

A parasagittal section is used for direct observation of the activation of the lumbar multifidus for facilitation purposes.[136] The ultrasound transducer is placed lateral to the spinous processes, allowing a longitudinal image of the multifidus, including the dysfunctional segment (Fig. 9.8). Particular interest should be centred on watching the deep fibres of the muscle adjacent to the zygapophyseal joints (Fig. 9.9). The patient can observe the muscle contraction while consciously trying to 'swell out' the muscle at the segmental level, or trying to activate the muscle with the contraction of the transversus abdominis or the pelvic floor. Simultaneously, the patient can palpate the lower abdomen to feel the transversus abdominis co-activation. Precise feedback is given, which ensures that the patient is activating the multifidus at the affected segment. The quality of the contraction is appreciated as a slow increase in vertical depth of the multifidus, including the deep fibres, and the ability to hold the contraction can also be monitored as the maintenance of this vertical dimension. The use of ultrasound imaging as a feedback tool in rehabilitation provides a notable advance in the rehabilitation of deep muscles, which cannot be viewed or palpated with any degree of certainty.

In practice, other external visual facilitatory techniques may be used, including the use of a mirror placed obliquely at the side of the patient so that he or she can monitor the appearance of the abdominal wall for their own practice at home. The provision of specific guidelines to the patient indicating the external appearance of the abdominal wall in their specific substitution strategy and how they may recognize this is vital. This visual feedback is best accompanied by palpation for either the gentle contraction in the lower abdomen or for deep tension development in the segmental multifidus (Fig. 9.10).

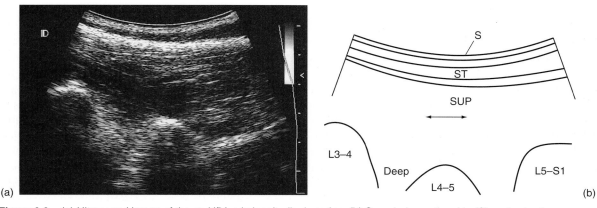

**Figure 9.9**    (a) Ultrasound image of the multifidus in longitudinal section. (b) Superiorly are the skin (S) and subcutaneous tissue (ST). The multifidus fibres run in the direction of the arrow (↔). Inferiorly are the zygapophyseal joints L3–L4, L4–L5 and L5–S1. The deep fibres of the multifidus are seen surrounding the zygapophyseal joints. Deep, deep multifidus fibres; SUP, superficial.

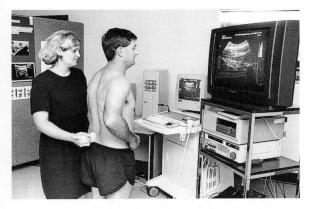

**Figure 9.10** Visual and tactile feedback for the patient when practising the deep muscle co-contraction.

In some cases, when the patient is performing the transversus abdominis or the lumbar multifidus contraction independently of the other trunk muscles, they may claim that they feel they are doing nothing. This is generally because the contraction is subtle, and the normal perception of an abdominal muscle contraction, for example, is the performance of a trunk movement such as a sit-up or posterior pelvic tilt. Verbal reassurance that this is normal and reiteration of the functional role of the muscles is always required. It also highlights the importance of the patient understanding the whole concept of deep muscle support and control, and points to the potential future more routine use of ultrasound imaging in rehabilitation.

### Lumbopelvic position

Although any of the techniques described above may be used in many different body positions, the precise position of the lumbopelvic region may itself be facilitatory for activation of the transversus abdominis or lumbar multifidus. In support of this relationship, we have some indication that pelvic floor muscle contraction can successfully isolate the transversus abdominis from the other abdominal muscles when the lumbar spine is placed in a more neutral position[298] (see Fig. 4.11, Ch. 4). There is a consensus that the local muscles are involved in segmental support and, therefore, contribute to the precise positioning of the lumbosacral curve. Thus positioning the spine in a precise neutral lumbosacral curve may be successful in assisting the patient to achieve a co-contraction of the transversus abdominis and lumbar multifidus.

Teaching the patient to assume an upright neutral posture in sitting or standing must be done with care and is the essential feature of this facilitation strategy.[124] The aim is for an upright position of the pelvis with restoration of a normal lumbosacral lordosis (Fig. 9.11a). If the patient has inadequate range of movement or pain with movement in the L4–L5 and L5–S1 segments, poor kinesthetic sense in their lower lumbar joints, poor local muscle control, or overactive thoracic portions of the erector spinae muscles, then the upright trunk position may be achieved by inappropriate extension in the thoracolumbar region (Fig. 9.11b). Treatment may need to be addressed initially towards reducing the pain and restoring segmental movement if hypomobility is the problem. To assume the upright, neutral postural position, correction should be initiated at the pelvis. Often the patient has poor awareness and it is usually necessary for them to have a tactile cue to locate the lumbosacral junction, and this most simply is their thumb or finger. Once in position, the patient then focuses on deep muscle activation using whichever strategy is most effective, whether via abdominal drawing in, activating the pelvic floor or isometrically setting the multifidus.

### Direct strategies to decrease overactivity of muscles

Many of the techniques already described incorporate body positions or strategies to decrease overactivity of global muscles. As mentioned, the muscles of primary concern with respect to overactivity are the oblique abdominal muscles. If the patient has difficulty relaxing these or other global muscles and the strategies already described are unsuccessful, then the clinician can explore other measures to gain relaxation of the overactive muscle(s).

**Restoration of normal breathing.** We have observed clinically that breathing patterns are

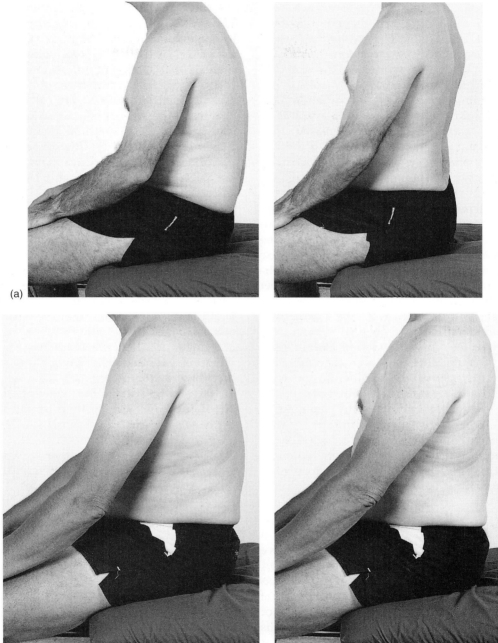

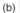

**Figure 9.11**    The upright neutral posture. (a) Left: relaxed sitting posture. Right: Normal lumbosacral position. (b) Left: relaxed sitting position. Right: the upright trunk position is attained through an incorrect extension in the thoracolumbar region, which leaves the lumbosacral junction in flexion.

sometimes altered in chronic low back pain patients. In normal inspiration, the most important muscle is the diaphragm. The abdominal muscles are not involved. In forced expiration, the abdominal muscles act both to depress the thoracic cage and to elevate the diaphragm by raising the intra-abdominal pressure.[82] The abdominal muscles should only take part in the respiratory cycle when expiratory flow is increased; they should remain relaxed in normal quiet breathing. One recent study has reported activation of the transversus abdominis, but not the global abdominal muscles, during relaxed breathing.[1]

In a small percentage of chronic low back pain patients, the activity of obliquus externus abdominis has been observed clinically during quiet inspiration and expiration. We have also observed the use of accessory muscles of inspiration in these patients, and patterns of upper chest breathing. The cause of this change in breathing pattern is not clear and is an area of ongoing research. A method of decreasing the activation of the obliquus externus abdominis is to teach the patient diaphragmatic breathing patterns. The use of positioning (as in postoperative and respiratory patients) should be remembered for patients who are having difficulty in establishing the appropriate relaxed breathing pattern. The reader is referred to respiratory physical therapy texts for the many alternatives.[107] As the patient learns to control the diaphragm, the muscles of the abdominal wall can relax, and co-contraction exercises can begin. If the obliquus externus abdominis is active in breathing, it is our experience that it will be challenging to facilitate an isolated contraction of the deep corset muscles.

**EMG biofeedback.** Biofeedback from EMG has traditionally been used on the target muscle of the rehabilitation exercise to provide evidence of its contraction.[315] In retraining the transversus abdominis, electrodes placed over the lateral abdominal wall will detect electromyographic activity from all muscles, and therefore provide little useful information. Placement of an electrode over the triangle formed between the anterior superior iliac spine, navel and pubic symphysis will detect the activity of both the obliquus

internus abdominis and the transversus abdominis, making this placement unsuitable when attempting to train a more isolated activation of the transversus abdominis. It also appears that EMG is of little value for providing feedback for the multifidus contraction. While the muscle becomes superficial in the lower regions of the lumbar spine, it is the deep fibres that are most involved in segmental support. Nevertheless, in the training of the deep muscle co-contraction, biofeedback from EMG has become a most successful adjunct to treatment. Instead of being used to monitor the activation in contracting muscles, it is used to ensure relaxation in the global muscles while training the independent activation of the deep muscles.

The use of biofeedback from EMG has proved particularly helpful in assisting patients to relax excessive activity and avoid substitution by the obliquus externus abdominis and the rectus abdominis, as well as the thoracic portions of the erector spinae (Fig. 9.12). The most appropriate placement for the electrodes for viewing the obliquus externus abdominis is in parallel with the fibres of this muscle over the anterior end of the eighth rib.[253] For viewing the rectus abdominis, the best position of the electrodes is below the navel, 2 cm lateral to the midline.

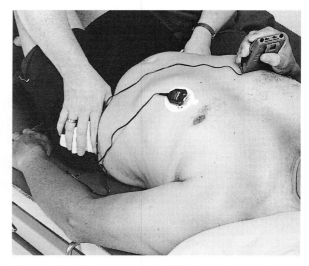

**Figure 9.12**   Placement of the EMG electrode over the eighth rib to monitor activity in the obliquus externus abdominis.

With these electrode positions there is minimal interference from the adjacent abdominal muscles. The biofeedback from EMG can be used in conjunction with all the other facilitation strategies discussed, and is used potently with feedback from ultrasound imaging. It is a method that is growing in use in the clinical situation due to its effectiveness in giving some objectivity to the effectiveness of the technique chosen.

For reasons identical to those described above, electrical stimulation is not an option when training isolated contraction of the transversus abdominis, since other muscles almost always overlie it.

**Elevation of the rib cage.** Since the action of obliquus externus abdominis on the rib cage is to draw the ribs downwards and inwards, it can be useful to cognitively use the intercostal muscles to elevate the rib cage prior to the performance of transversus abdominis contraction in an attempt to reduce obliquus externus abdominis substitution. To implement this technique, the therapist instructs the patient to perform a gentle bibasal expansion against either the therapist's or their own hands placed laterally on the rib cage. Once this has been performed the patient then performs a contraction of the transversus abdominis, either directly or using one of the other facilitation techniques such as pelvic floor muscle contraction. It is essential that the therapist assesses and ensures that the rib cage elevation has been successful in reducing obliquus externus abdominis contraction before the transversus abdominis contraction is attempted. If not, another technique should be tried. Other techniques of assisting the bibasal expansion can be used, such as a belt placed around the lower rib cage. An alternative technique involves placing the hands behind the head with the elbows stretched laterally in order to passively elevate the rib cage. The emphasis at all times is on the use of minimal effort to produce the rib cage elevation, in order to avoid activation of the other global muscles.

**Other inhibitory techniques and positions.** For those skilled in them, there are many different techniques within physical therapy practice that can be used to decrease overactivity in muscles, and notably in this case the obliquus externus abdominis. Various neurological techniques such as proprioceptive neuromuscular facilitation[189] and Bobath techniques[208] provide useful methods of addressing the problems of overactive muscles. Other techniques such as myofascial treatment of the abdominal and lumbar trigger points[335] or deep inhibitory massage may also be appropriate to achieve relaxation. Taping techniques may also be of use.

## IMPLEMENTATION OF THE ACTIVATION STRATEGIES

Many different techniques are available to assist in the facilitation of transversus abdominis and lumbar multifidus activation. Those described here are by no means all of them, and many additional techniques may exist that achieve the same goal. The clinician should keep in mind that the goal of the procedure is to isolate the contraction of the transversus abdominis and lumbar multifidus so that the ability of these muscles to contract can be improved. The possibilities for facilitation are limited only by the creativity of the clinician. When trialling alternative techniques it is essential to monitor closely for the appearance of substitution strategies. It is also important to remember that no one technique works for all people, and the clinician must keep aware of what is occurring so that a technique is quickly discarded if it is unsuccessful and another technique tried.

Each of the techniques described can be used in combination as well as separately. The clinician should be willing to try many different combinations until he or she is satisfied that the patient has achieved the best contraction. At first the clinician may find this time-consuming, but with practice and experience it is possible to identify patient presentations which suggest that a particular technique or combination of techniques may be the most appropriate. Logically, the most rapid rate of improvement can be expected if the best facilitation technique is identified for that patient.

Once a method has been found which results in contraction of the transversus abdominis and lumbar multifidus in relative isolation from the global trunk muscles, the effectiveness of the contraction is enhanced by repetition of the contraction. It is imperative that the patient can undertake the facilitation technique independently so that it can be practised at home between treatment sessions. In this phase of motor relearning, repetition is key, and the clinician and patient should plan times for practice. Furthermore, for motor relearning to be effective, it is imperative that the patient is repeating the correct action. The initial home programme must be clearly taught and documented so that both parties are confident that the programme is achievable. It is very useful to show patients strategies of self-detection of substitutions. Self-palpation of the abdomen medial to the anterior superior iliac crest can be used, with the patient instructed to avoid pushing out against their fingers, indicating an incorrect pattern of activation. The home programme should be tested in full at all treatment sessions with respect to the specific position, number of repetitions and contraction holding times. As soon as possible, the patient needs to be taught and be able to achieve the deep muscle co-contraction in many different postures, particularly standing and sitting (Fig. 9.13). This makes frequent practice more convenient and allows it to be incorporated into daily activities without too much disruption to lifestyle. Greater convenience of practice increases compliance.

It is essential that clinicians ask themselves three central questions before they permit a patient to go home to practice. These are:

- What strategy works best to isolate the contraction of the transversus abdominis or lumbar multifidus from contraction of the global muscles?
- How can the clinician and patient be sure that the correct contraction will be performed at home in each practice period?
- How many contractions can be performed? How long can a contraction be held before it is lost or another muscle has been substituted?

One of the main advantages of the patient being able to self-assess for substitutions or loss of holding is that they can to a certain extent self-

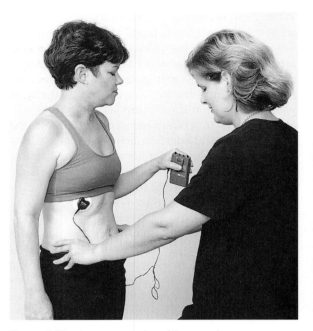

**Figure 9.13** As a progression of the exercise programme the deep muscle co-contraction is taught in standing. Note that biofeedback from EMG is useful for this patient, whose oblique abdominals are overactive in this position.

direct progression by increasing the duration and number of contractions as their ability to activate the muscles improves.

It is necessary to assess that the technique chosen has successfully changed the ability of the patient to perform the muscle contraction. While palpation can be used as a cue for the activation of the transversus abdominis, it is not reliable as a means of quantitative assessment. The only means available in the clinical situation to be assured that the deep muscle co-contraction is improving is to regularly repeat the prone test using the pressure biofeedback unit. In the initial stages of activation, the deep muscle may not be able to generate enough force to draw in the abdominal wall to reduce pressure.

Rechecks at regular intervals should show the patient gradually being able to reduce pressure by greater magnitudes as the activation and quality of contraction improve with the chosen exercise strategies. It is important to remember that a decrease in substitution by the global muscles (i.e. an improvement in pattern) also constitutes an improvement in the clinical test, especially in the initial stage.

The length of time of this stage is variable and depends on the degree of a patient's motor control problems as well as their motivation and enthusiasm to practise. In controlled clinical trials, it has been demonstrated that this stage could be as long as 6–10 weeks in chronic patients,[257,259] whereas in acute first-episode low back pain patients recovery was achieved within 2–3 weeks.[136] (see Box 9.4.)

---

**Box 9.4**   The formal training of the motor skill of deep muscle co-contraction

- Analyse the unwanted global muscle overactivity.
- Improve the perception of the deep muscle co-contraction.
- Select individual strategies to improve the precision of the co-contraction.
- Repeated practice.
- Control of the skill in functional upright positions.
- Quantitatively re-evaluate the skill (prone test)

# 10

# Integration into dynamic function

Once the patient can perform a voluntary co-contraction of the transversus abdominis and lumbar multifidus independently of the global muscles, and can hold this contraction in any position or posture, the aim of treatment is the integration of the motor skill into normal static and dynamic functional tasks. Progress is made by incorporating the motor skill into light functional tasks, with gradual progress to heavy-load functional tasks as required by the individual patient. It is important to remember that the global muscles are essential for controlling external loading and spinal orientation (see Ch. 2), while the local muscles provide segmental control. Thus, a main aim of this progression of treatment is to teach the patient to overlay contraction of the global muscles onto the local muscle contraction in a functionally appropriate way that does not compromise or promote complete substitution for the action of the local muscle system.

## INCORPORATION OF THE MOTOR SKILL INTO LIGHT FUNCTIONAL TASKS

This stage aims to continue to train the deep muscle co-contraction with the added challenge of light loads. At this level, the deep muscle co-contraction is trained in the presence of activity of the global muscle system while normal breathing patterns are able to be continued. That is, activities which may need breath-holding and the valsalva manoeuvre as in heavy lifting would not be emphasized at this stage of training of the deep muscles. Two functional conditions are trained. The first requires the deep muscles to maintain their lumbopelvic supporting function in static conditions under light load in concert with the muscles of the global system, while breathing normally. The second requires the deep muscles to maintain their lumbopelvic supporting function during trunk movement around the neutral position, while the muscles of the global system are acting phasically (i.e. out of concert with the type of contraction being performed by the deep local system). Again, normal breathing patterns are maintained in these conditions.

A third functional condition requires the performance of the co-contraction in postures or during moving to control positions that normally aggravate the pain. These represent quite high levels of difficulty for training control of the deep mucle system. As for the formal motor skill training, the emphasis is on precision and control, as the deep and global muscle systems are now being trained in their interdependent and independent roles.

## Control of neutral lumbopelvic postures

Patients have now been trained to hold the deep muscle contraction in sitting and standing postures. They now begin to hold this contraction and maintain pelvic control, while undertaking activities where the upper and lower limbs are taking part in functional tasks, for example while sitting and working on a computer, reaching for documents or driving a car (although, safety first!). In many cases, the clinician may find a more formal approach to this part of training is more beneficial, as it allows the patients to become more involved in their progress on a day-to-day basis. Future research is required to investigate if the effects of formal training are transferred to the functional situation. At this time the more formal training used involves either low level leg-loading exercises in supine lying, or trunk inclination tasks, which are usually performed in sitting. As both exercises require static trunk positions, it is important for the clinician to keep

in mind the potential problems of trunk rigidity if this stage of training is taken to the extreme.

### Leg loading

In the first instance, the local and global muscle systems may be challenged by external loads via leg-loading exercises. The exercises described here are based on the concept of leg loading for lumbopelvic control described by Sahrmann[294,295] and White & Sahrmann.[353] Beginning with leg-loading exercises has several advantages. As mentioned, both the local and global systems are working synergistically in common in a static supporting role. Additionally, the magnitude of resistance can be controlled, and successful maintenance of control of trunk position can be monitored objectively using the pressure biofeedback unit, which gives immediate feedback of any change in lumbopelvic position. The way in which steady pressure readings (on 40 mmHg) can be used to indicate lumbopelvic control should be explained to the patient (Fig. 10.1). For details on the use of the biofeedback unit, see the Appendix to Chapter 8.

Training can proceed from the level formally assessed for the individual patient (Ch. 8). Most often this means that training begins at very low levels of load. One of the most telling factors resulting from the objective feedback provided by the use of the pressure biofeedback unit is the previous tendency for patients to be trained at

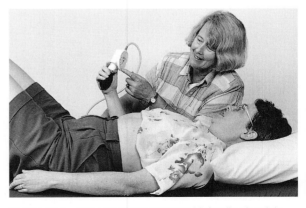

**Figure 10.1**   The use of the pressure biofeedback unit is explained to the patient.

loads far in excess of that which they could control. At this stage, training is restricted to the crook lying position and to unilateral leg loading, the moving leg maintaining contact with the exercise surface in order to lessen the level of load to less than leg weight. The other leg provides some passive stability and remains supported. With the leg moving into abduction and external rotation, the patient focuses on learning rotatory control of the lumbopelvic region (Fig. 10.2), while straightening the leg to an extended abduction position adds a sagittal plane control component (Fig. 10.3). For both directions of loading, the pressure biofeedback unit is placed longitudinally adjacent the spine in order better to monitor any unwanted trunk rotation or extension. Once in position, it is inflated to 40 mmHg.

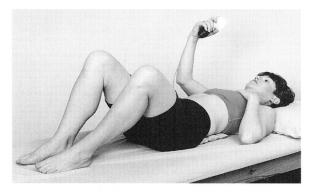

**Figure 10.2**  Training rotatory control with light leg load.

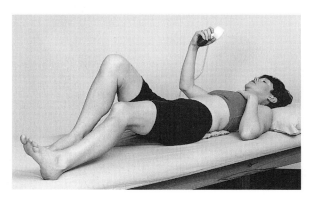

**Figure 10.3**  Training more complex control with supported leg extension or abduction.

Exercises are performed with a common proforma. First, the patient draws in the abdominal wall in order to consciously activate the transversus abdominis and lumbar multifidus. This co-contraction must be held throughout the entire leg-loading manoeuvre, while also maintaining a normal breathing pattern. The leg must be moved slowly, with the emphasis being on precision and control. The patient only moves the leg to positions in which the lumbopelvic position can be maintained. Control is defined by the two parameters that are monitored in formal testing. There should be no change in pressure registered on the pressure biofeedback unit, as this signals loss of control of lumbopelvic position. The abdominal wall needs to remain flat during the entire exercise, as this is likely to indicate that the transversus abdominis is coping with the imposed load.[242] If the abdominal wall bulges, it is probable that the load has exceeded the capacity of the transversus abdominis and it has lost its corset-like contraction. Exercise repetition may be low in the early stages, as the muscles can fatigue quite readily. Progression is through increased repetition, and movement of the limb through its full excursion.

Muscle lengthening procedures for muscles attaching to the lumbar spine and pelvis offer

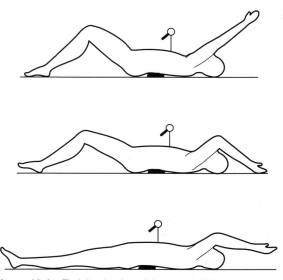

**Figure 10.4**  Training lumbopelvic control during lengthening of the latissimus dorsi.

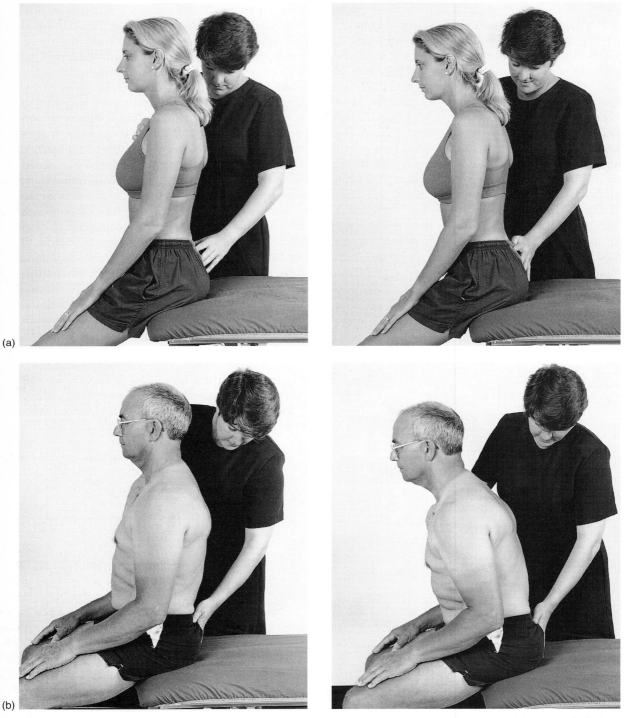

(a)

(b)

**Figure 10.5** (a) (Left) Sitting in the correct upright neutral posture; (right) Control of the neutral lumbopelvic posture in flexion (b) (Left) Sitting in the upright posture; (right) loss of control of the neutral lumbopelvic posture in flexion.

the same challenges to the maintainance of lumbopelvic stability. In addition, some muscles of the global system with attachments to the lumbar spine, such as the latissimus dorsi and iliopsoas, must be able to lengthen without compromising the stability of the region (see Ch. 2). The precision and monitoring of progression used for the leg-loading exercises are equally applicable to muscle lengthening procedures (Fig. 10 4).

### Trunk inclination exercises

Intrinsic loads can be placed on the deep muscle co-contraction to train its force-generating and endurance abilities. This is done by requiring patients to control and hold a neutral upright lumbopelvic posture during forward trunk inclination with hip flexion.[124,188] Small trunk inclinations are used, starting at 5° and progressing to 10° and then 15°; this is in line with the aim to train at low loads. The subject first attains the correct upright neutral posture (Fig. 10.5a, left), and activates the deep muscle co-contraction. The key to this exercise is for the patient to maintain control of the lumbosacral curve with the deep muscles during the trunk inclination (Fig. 10.5a, right). Loss of control can be monitored by viewing or palpating a subtle movement of the low lumbar segments into flexion and a simultaneous subtle increase in the activity of the thoracic portions of the erector spinae, which encourage the formation of a lordosis (or extension) in the thoracolumbar region (Fig. 10.5b). The exercise is first practised in sitting, but it can also be undertaken in standing. This exercise is similar to the waiter's bow exercise described by Sahrmann.[294,295]

## Lumbopelvic control during trunk movement

Normal function requires that the deep muscles can maintain continuous tonic activity to support the lumbar segments and lumbopelvic region, while muscles of the global system work phasically to produce or control total trunk movement and orientation. With the knowledge that the transversus abdominis, in its dysfunc-

tional state in low back pain patients, loses this separate control from the muscles of the global system,[146,148] retraining this separate control using directly opposite functions of the local and global systems is challenging. Walking provides an ideal fundamental human function in which patients can train this capacity. As a prerequisite to this stage, the patient must be able to activate the transversus abdominis and lumbar multifidus independently of the global muscles. The patient's task in this phase is to activate and hold the deep muscle co-contraction and then to slowly practise walking while concentrating on maintaining the contraction (Fig. 10.6). This exercise is often quite fatiguing in the early attempts, and care must be taken that the patient does not switch to a global muscle substitution. As a progression, the patient increases the distance walked while consciously controlling the deep muscle activation, and then increases the speed of walking. As mentioned, gait is a fundamental human function, and this exercise not

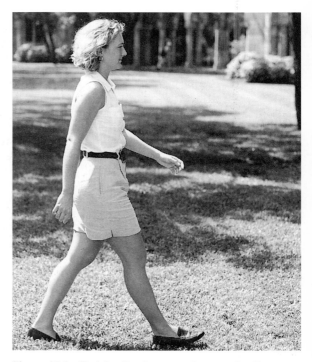

**Figure 10.6**   Training the deep muscle co-contraction during walking.

only serves as a convenient format for patients to practise towards automatic control, but it is also a function in which automatic activation of the deep muscles is deemed essential.[54]

Deep muscle control is also trained through the range of spinal movement. The transversus abdominis and lumbar multifidus are activated in upright standing, and the patient learns to hold the contraction while slowly moving through the conventional planes of motion. Control of pain in an otherwise painful direction of movement is a powerful illustrator of the effect of muscle support, and offers the patient a powerful incentive to practise. As well as the pure planes of motion, training can be extended to combined planes, particularly those combinations of movement that are usually pain provoking and problematic (Fig. 10.7). Such techniques were successfully used by O'Sullivan et al[257] in their management of patients with spondylolysis and spondylolisthesis.

Critical evaluation of the effectiveness of a particular technique or regime is an important element of management. As the patient trains the co-contraction of the deep muscles under different conditions throughout this stage, it is always necessary to reassess the quality of the contrac-

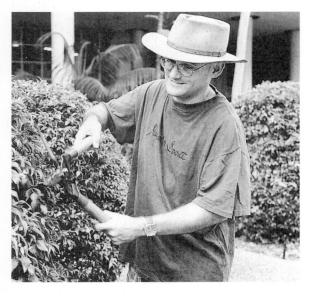

**Figure 10.7** Training the deep muscle co-contraction in a position/task which is usually problematic.

tion and the patient's ability to hold the contraction. This is done by returning to the formal prone test of the abdominal drawing-in action, using the pressure biofeedback unit. This objectivity is needed, as visual inspection and palpation of the lower abdominal wall are insufficient, unreliable and can be misleading.

## INCORPORATION OF THE MOTOR SKILL INTO HEAVIER FUNCTIONAL TASKS

This next stage of the programme aims to ensure that the contraction and holding ability of the transversus abdominis and multifidus are sufficient to control lumbar spine position with increasing loads. The level of load required depends on the individual patient, and must match the needs and requirements of the patient's work and lifestyle. It consists of formal exercise training programmes and functional exercise programmes related to the patient's daily living activities, work and sport.

### Formal exercise programmes

Load is gradually added to the system through a variety of exercises. The spine is controlled in a neutral position. Many of these more general exercises have features in common with other exercise programmes.[101,288,293–295,353] Load can be applied through body positioning, challenging the muscle system by decreasing the stability of the body position, use of equipment or the direct application of increasing load.

There are some basic elements in common to all the exercises at this stage. The performance of any exercise must be preceded by a conscious activation of the deep muscles by gently drawing in the abdomen. The abdominal wall must remain flat during the exercise and not bulge (bulging suggests that the transversus abdominis corset-like contraction has been lost). The emphasis is still on control, and progression should not be too fast, as too much load too quickly may lead to the global muscles coping uniquely with the load with loss of support to the spinal segments. Regular reassessment of the local muscle performance must be done using the prone abdominal drawing-in test. In addition, the capacity of the system under load is monitored using formal leg-loading tests and the pressure biofeedback unit.

Several different exercises have been tested for their suitability to encourage a co-contraction of the trunk flexors and extensors in order to enhance general trunk stability.[285] Exercises that induce a rotatory load on to the trunk are particularly appropriate. The four-point kneeling position offers a good starting position to link the training of the initial stage with this stage of added load.

First, the patient is taught precision in positioning, as often the posture in four-point kneeling is poor, and the whole thoracolumbar spine is flexed or in a kyphosis, or the low lumbar area is kyphotic with the lordosis in the lower thoracic upper lumbar areas. Such postures may reflect dominant activity in the thoracic portions of erector spinae and the obliquus externus abdominis and rectus abdominis (Fig. 10.8). To obtain a good posture, the knees are positioned under the hips, and the hands under the shoulders, and the actions of several deep and postural muscles are recruited.

Any overactivity, in particular in the obliquus externus abdominis, should be addressed first and the patient encouraged to relax this muscle. The lumbosacral spine is positioned in neutral to obtain a correct posture of the whole spine up to the craniocervical region. To achieve this, the lower portions of the lumbar multifidus are recruited to obtain a normal lumbosacral lordosis; the lower trapezius and serratus anterior in particular are used to obtain a correct posture of the thoracic spine and scapulae. This is achieved by letting the patient 'hang' their thoracic spine between their shoulder blades, and then actively protracting their scapulae while gently drawing up their thoracic spine through the action of the serratus anterior. The common fault to be corrected is use of the obliquus externus abdominis and rectus abdominis as a substitute, this being recognizable as thoracolumbar flexion. The head posture should be in neutral alignment. An active support of this posture is often chal-

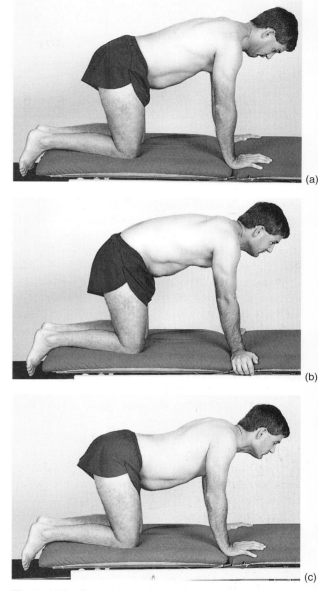

(a)

(b)

(c)

**Figure 10.8**   Posture in the four-point kneeling position: (a) correct postural position; (b) a flexed spinal posture; (c) a reversal of normal thoracolumbar posture.

lenging for the low back pain patient and, in the first instance, they may merely need to practise assuming and holding this posture.

A rotatory load is applied to the trunk muscle system by extending the opposite arm and leg to

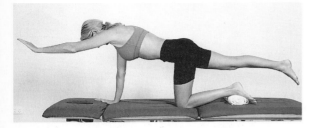

**Figure 10.9**  Four-point kneeling with arm and leg extension. The patient controls the neutral spinal posture and pelvic position.

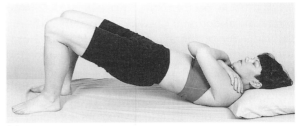

(a)

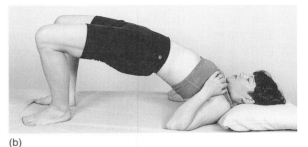

(b)

**Figure 10.10**  (a) Bridging, while holding the spine in a neutral position. (b) Incorrect bridging, with the spine in an extended position.

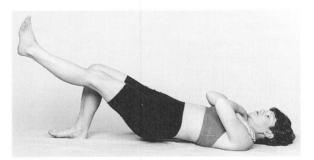

**Figure 10.11**  The bridging exercise with single leg extension. Done correctly, the exercise challenges the stabilizing system of the lumbopelvic area. Note the lumbopelvic flexion and rotation, which indicate that this exercise is too difficult for this patient.

a horizontal position (Fig. 10.9). The exercise can be performed poorly and ineffectively if precision is not emphasized. The patient should first activate the deep muscles by drawing in the lower abdominal wall and holding this contraction throughout the exercise. The leg is slowly extended, the patient focusing not on lifting the leg but on maintaining the lumbopelvic position (not allowing the pelvis to lift or dip into rotation or hyperextension). When controlling this position, the arm is raised, with a similar focus on trunk and girdle control. The position is held for up to 5 s and the exercise is then repeated using the opposite diagonal. The exercise can be progressed by challenging trunk stability through the principle of unstable surfaces. A ball or small balance board can be placed under the supporting hand and the patient works to maintain the contraction of the deep muscles and a steady trunk position.

Bridging from the crook lying position can be used as a basic exercise and position. Again, care must be taken with performance to gain value from the exercise. Prior to the bridge, the deep muscle co-contraction is performed and the patient bridges, focusing on lifting the pelvis and extending the hips with a gluteal contraction, keeping the spine in a neutral position. This position and a common fault are shown in Figure 10.10. Direct rotatory resistance can be applied to the pelvis by the clinician and subsequently by the patient. The resistance can be applied slowly in the form of alternating isometrics,[326] with each contraction being held for 5 s.

The bridging exercise can be advanced by decreasing the base of support through single leg extension (Fig. 10.11), with the emphasis on keeping the trunk and pelvis steady. Again, the task can be made even more difficult by making the supporting surface unstable by placing a ball under the foot. An alternative progression is to introduce the element of speed, which challenges the global muscles to be working phasically

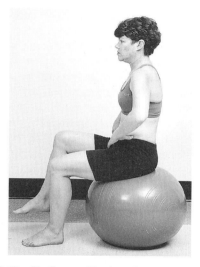

**Figure 10.12**    Challenge of lumbopelvic control in sitting by using a gym ball as the supporting surface.

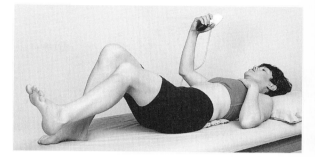

**Figure 10.13**    Leg-loading exercise with unsupported extension of one leg. The pressure must be maintained without fluctuations and the abdominal wall must remain flat.

while the deep muscles hold their isometric contraction. The patient focuses on keeping the abdomen flat and pelvis steady while rhythmically extending alternate legs. This is done slowly at first; as the patient gains control, the speed of the alternate leg can be increased gradually.[326]

The principle of unstable surfaces can be incorporated into many different exercise programmes. Good use can be made of large gym balls, and several exercises and general stabilization programmes have been described illustrating their use.[188,288] Sitting postural control can be challenged (Fig. 10.12), and any of the bridging and exercises in four-point kneeling can be made more difficult by using a ball as a supporting surface.

Leg-loading exercises can be advanced from those practised in the previous stage. The load should be increased slowly, and control of the lumbopelvic region monitored using the pressure biofeedback unit. This feedback helps ensure precision in the exercise and guides logical progression. At all times the exercise is preceded by a deep muscle co-contraction and, as before, the abdomen should remain flat throughout the exercise. Progression can proceed from single leg supported extension (the leg moving into extension and abduction to incorporate a rotatory

load), to single leg unsupported extension (Fig. 10.13). For patients requiring high strength, the exercise can be advanced to double leg extension. The clinician will note that the patient's normal breathing pattern is challenged as the work required by the global muscles increases.

Muscle lengthening procedures for the lower limb can induce high loads onto the lumbar spine, and stretching techniques must be designed with lumbopelvic stability in mind (Fig. 10.14). Obviously, it is important to avoid injury to the lumbar spine during training.

At regular intervals throughout the training programme with load, the capacity of the transversus abdominis and lumbar multifidus must be formally tested using the prone abdominal drawing-in test, in order to ensure that the global muscle system is not being trained at the expense of the local muscle system. This is particularly so for patients who have demonstrated marked overactivity in the obliquus externus abdominis, who may revert to poor strategies and patterns if not monitored closely at all stages. The effect of exercise on the interaction between the local and global muscle systems is monitored using the leg-loading tests and the pressure biofeedback unit.

## Functional exercise programmes

Functional exercise programmes relevant to the patient's activities of daily living, work and sport constitute the final stage of rehabilitation. Training for deep muscle support during high-

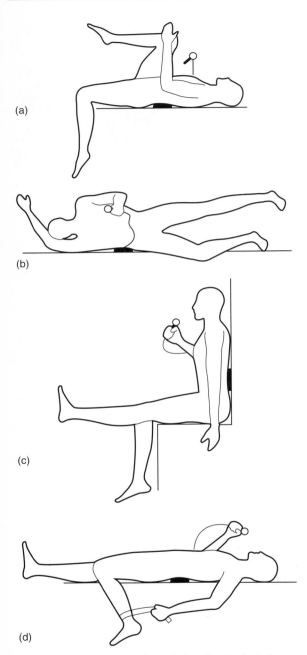

**Figure 10.14** Examples of muscle lengthening techniques in which lumbar spine stability must be monitored: (a) iliopsoas; (b) tensor fasciae latae; (c) hamstrings; (d) rectus femoris.

impact loading activities such as running and jumping may need to be incorporated into the rehabilitation programme. Teaching practices of safe lifting, carrying and handling, or the correction of styles in sport, are integral components of all rehabilitation programmes, and many of the correct practices are integrated into the patient management early in the programme but practised without load. McGill & Norman[224] have developed provisional guidelines for lifting based on world-wide biomechanical research and the developing knowledge of muscle function in stabilization of the spine. They identify the need to 'lightly co-contract the stabilizing musculature to remove the slack from the system and stiffen the spine' as one of the criteria for safe lifting (Box 10.1). Our research has supported this need and has provided more specific information about which specific muscles are needed to provide segmental support. Even more importantly, our research has shown that the deep muscles designed to stiffen the spinal segments for safe lifting are those which become dysfunctional in low back pain. Safe lifting will only proceed if the deep muscles are effectively and specifically rehabilitated.

There is no argument that functional ability is

---

**Box 10.1** Summary of McGill & Norman's provisional guidelines for lifting*

- Maintain normal lordosis and rotate the trunk using the hips.
- Allow time for the disc nucleus to equilibrate and the ligaments to regain stiffness after prolonged flexion.
- Avoid lifting shortly after arising from bed.
- *Lightly co-contract the stabilizing musculature to remove the slack from the system and stiffen the spine.*
- Choose a posture to minimize the reaction moment on the back, but do not compromise the maintenance of the normal lordosis.
- Avoid twisting.
- Exploit the acceleration profile of the load.

*Adapted from McGill & Norman,[224] p. 112.

an ultimate goal of rehabilitation in association with relief of pain and prevention of recurrent episodes. Persons must be trained to cope with the loads inherent in their daily activities, work practices or sport. What must be ensured is that the deep muscle system is trained to supply the inner support so that forces absorbed by the global muscles in high or rapid loading can be transferred safely and efficiently to the passive structures. At the present time there are no methods for checking if appropriate control of segmental motion is occurring during functional tasks. The assessment of deep muscle activation and holding ability introduced in this text (see Ch. 8) remain the only objective measures available at this time. Research to indicate whether these tests reflect automatic deep muscle function in complex functional activities or indeed research to develop measures capable of demonstrating if problems do exist in the deep muscles during such activities, present the ultimate challenge of this approach to the treatment of motor-control problems in the deep muscles of low back pain patients.

# 11

# Practical aspects of treatment planning and delivery

Clinicians are faced with a variety of low back pain patients presenting with different pathologies and problems, ranging from those suffering their first episode of low back pain to those with chronic and persistent back pain. The physical presentation of back pain patients is also highly variable, ranging from an acute pain state with a marked deformity and grossly limited active movements, to the situation where pain is not severe but is persistent, and active movements are relatively pain-free. Confronted with this diversity, there are three very legitimate questions that are often asked by clinicians:

- Which patients require stabilization training?
- Are other treatments used in the management of low back pain patients still relevant?
- When can stabilization training begin?

## TREATMENT PLANNING

### Stabilization training

When deciding whether a patient needs stabilization training there are two issues to consider. Current evidence suggests that the problems which present in the deep or local muscles of the lumbopelvic region are not pathology specific. To date, a variety of back pain patients have been studied in the clinic and laboratory. Some patients had evident morphological change, but often the diagnosis was non-specific mechanical low back pain. The impairments in the deep muscles characterize back pain patients, and this is independent of the likely variety in pathology in these subjects.[136,139,146,257,259,282] This finding is not surprising and is consistent with the fairly regular reactions observed in muscles with primary antigravity and supporting functions in other regions of the body. For example, inhibition and wasting of the vastus medialis obliquus is inevitably present and indeed is pathognomonic of a problem in the knee, regardless of whether the patient has an acute anterior cruciate ligament rupture, an osteoarthritic knee or a patellofemoral complex problem. Therefore, it can be argued that all patients with low back pain potentially require assessment and retraining of their local muscle systems, just as all patients with knee joint arthropathies require specific quadriceps retraining. While pain may ease after an acute bout of back pain, there is no guarantee that the muscle will automatically recover. Indeed, evidence points to a lack of automatic recovery, despite a return to normal activity levels.[136]

The second issue involved in which patients require stabilization training revolves around terminology and concepts and definitions of clinical instability (see Ch. 2). Too often a very narrow definition of instability is applied, which focuses on the more major losses in integrity in the osseoligamentous system. It is well known that patients with a spondylolysis or spondylolisthesis or those with marked disc disruption have an instability problem. However, clinical stability as has been presented throughout this text is a broader issue, encompassing lack of proper functioning in any or all of the spinal stability systems, the passive or osseoligamentous subsystem, the active subsystem (the spinal muscles) and the neural control system.[262,263] Deficits in motor control in the deep, local muscle system have been shown in back pain patients with potentially different articular problems, and this suggests that clinical instability in its broader definition is a basic and fundamental impairment in back disability. Retraining motor control of the deep muscle system is required to redress a specific physical or neurophysiological impairment which is present in patients with low back pain and injury.

## Other treatments

From a physical perspective, back pain reflects a problem in a highly interrelated neuromuscular–articular system. No structure is necessarily spared from injury, and all structures of the motion segment are potential sources of pain. All systems and their reactions require attention in a comprehensive treatment programme. Other treatment strategies are still required for the patient with low back pain, and retraining the motor control of the deep muscles should be incorporated within a total management programme for the low back pain patient. This training is complementary to other management procedures, which are directed towards relieving pain, addressing other physical impairments inherent in the condition and restoring the patient to normal functional levels.

The other physical impairments in the articular or neural systems may be influencing the patient's ability to activate their deep muscles or be increasing the difficulty for the local muscles to provide segmental support. Joint injury and pain are well known to have profound effects on the muscle system. Relief of pain and restoration of motion and joint kinesthesia are fundamentally important to rehabilitation, not only of the segmental joint complex,[156] but also of the muscle system itself. As such, manipulative therapy is still very much indicated to relieve pain and restore segmental joint motion, and is usually an important component of total patient management. Retraining muscle control of the spinal segment is complementary to both passive manipulative therapy procedures and active joint mobilization, and all treatments can be commenced together with quite distinct but interrelated treatment rationales.

Restrictions in range or movement abnormalities in adjacent spinal, pelvic or hip joints are not infrequently a feature in the physical presentation of low back pain patients. When motion deficits in adjacent joints cause compensatory increases in or altered motion at the lumbosacral area, it may become more difficult for the muscles to maintain lumbopelvic support. Similarly, overactive or tight multijoint muscles in the lumbopelvic region, such as the quadratus lumborum, tensor fascia lata and hamstrings, can influence movement and control of the lumbar segments, and can reflect quite complex forces on the lumbar spine if their tightness is asymmetrical. These factors need to be addressed in the total management of the patient in order to optimize the environment for deep muscle retraining and function.

While there has been a deliberate focus on the deep muscle system in this text, this is not meant to detract from the importance of the global muscle system. Rather, such a focus reflects the fact that the global muscle system has already received copious attention in research and clinical practice. These muscles must be strong enough to take the external loads and protect the local muscle system and spinal segments by minimizing the loads on the lumbosacral region. Equally, their coordination must be efficient, in order to cope with and protect the spine from impact and other complex loading. In addition, low back pain sufferers may become deconditioned for the physical requirements of their lifestyles if their pain has been persistent and has decreased their overall activity levels. Such patients often eventually require cardiovascular and general exercise aimed at restoring fitness levels as needed for their work, sport or recreational demands.

## When can stabilization training begin?

Stabilization training can and should begin as early as possible in the patient's management, and there are few reasons why it should not be begun in the first treatment session in association with other treatment methods, which may be more focused on joint or neural tissue pain and dysfunction. Again, using the knee joint as an analogy, facilitation of the quadriceps is a routine part of an initial treatment of all knee conditions, regardless of other treatments employed. Nevertheless, in the early phases of rehabilitation of the patient with low back pain, care must be taken not to unduly stress recently injured and inflamed tissues,[43] as provocation of

pain during the exercise could cause further inhibition and should be avoided. The testing and facilitation of the transversus abdominis and the segmental lumbar multifidus are low-load procedures, with the patient positioned in a painless recumbent position, which should not compromise any damaged tissue. Furthermore, the spine is in a neutral posture; it has been shown that, even when joints are inflamed, in this posture the activation of articular nociceptors is minimal.[301] It must always be appreciated that the peripheral nociceptive sources and causes of back pain are the result of a complex interaction of factors. As much as manipulative therapy, electrophysical agents and medication may be prescribed to address and lessen the perception of pain, muscle control is a powerful factor which will assist in pain control.

Logically, muscle support should be restored to the spinal segment as soon as possible. As demonstrated in our study of first-episode acute low back pain patients,[136] early institution of methods to activate the deep muscles was not harmful with regard to resolution of painful symptoms when they were limited to low-load isometric exercise. In fact, far from being detrimental, the exercise was essential in preventing continuing reflex inhibition in the multifidus, which was still present at 10 weeks in the non-exercise group.

## TREATMENT DELIVERY

A basic proforma has been advocated throughout this text, i.e. to address motor control problems and then work towards restoration of trunk muscle stability capacity. The initial focus should be on training the motor skill by isolating the contraction of the deep muscles of the local system. The muscles must be trained so that they can be activated voluntarily by the patient and the patient can hold a low level isometric or tonic contraction repeatedly at will. A basic guideline for the patient is to aim ultimately to be able to hold a contraction for 10 s and be able to repeat this 10 times. Activation of the deep muscles can be incorporated into functional activities and, once the patient can activate and control the inner muscle unit, training of the outer muscle unit can begin safely and effectually. This involves first training the interaction between the outer and inner muscle layers in light functional tasks. Functional training under heavier loads can be introduced later in the programme to suit the level of a patient's work, sport and lifestyle demands. The ultimate aim is to restore the automatic (involuntary) protective function of the deep muscles without the need for voluntary activation of these muscles during functional tasks. In the clinical situation, it is difficult to predict whether this has occurred and, if so, whether it is permanent. For this reason, at present patients are usually requested to prophylactically practise the deep muscle co-contraction as part of a daily health routine, akin to cleaning their teeth every day. Only future prospective research will show whether the autonomic protective function is restored by training.

## Explaining the concept

Patients' concepts of exercise are usually more aligned to exercise for cardiovascular fitness, stretching and strength training. Thus asking them to perform the low-load precision exercises to activate the deep local muscles as a primary focus of the initial exercise programme is foreign to them. It is necessary, therefore, to carefully explain the nature and purpose of training a specific motor skill for joint stabilization, especially in the early stages of the programme.

It is wise to initially join their concept of exercise, and carefully explain the different forms of exercise training and their purposes. Patients understand well that if they wish to improve their cardiovascular fitness then they must undertake exercises such as walking, jogging, aerobics, cycling or swimming. They know that exercises to build up muscle strength often involve the use of weights. Motor skill training for spinal stabilization needs to be introduced as another form of exercise that is different to these more conventional and well-known exercise methods but vital to the alleviation and prevention of back pain.

To explain the concept of assessment and training the deep muscles for their function of joint control and support, it is important for the patient to understand the role of the deep muscles in normal function and in dysfunction. Several different examples can be given. Comparing the spine to a multisegmented flagpole is often a clear example. The long muscles of the trunk, such as the rectus abdominis and the thoraco-lumbar extensors, can be likened to the guy ropes that balance the whole pole while the deep muscles provide the link and support between each segment of the pole. It is of little use having strong guy ropes if there are weaknesses in the links between the segments; the pole will break at its weakest point, the injured lumbar inter-vertebral segment (Fig.11.1). Another strategy that is particularly helpful in getting the patient to visualize the role of the transversus abdominis in lumbar spine stabilization is to liken the spine, devoid of any muscles, to a piece of paper. If a force or load is applied to the single sheet, it will buckle. However, if the piece of paper is made into a cylinder by the transversus abdominis with the diaphragm as the lid and the pelvic floor as the base, it can now resist a force quite effectively. This is a very easy and convincing demonstration for the patient. Other patients may better visualize the role of the transversus abdominis and the deep back muscles as a deep muscle corset, which provides support and protects the injured joint in the back.

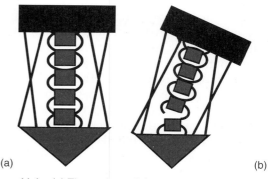

(a)                                                    (b)

**Figure 11.1**   (a) The analogy of the spine to a multisegmented flagpole supported by guy ropes and segmental links. (b) Despite strong guy ropes, the flagpole will become unstable if a segmental link is broken.

Research has provided evidence that the transversus abdominis and the lumbar multifidus are usually dysfunctional in low back pain patients. This will be reinforced by the assessment of these muscles using quantitative methods such as the use of the pressure biofeedback unit. It is a potent incentive to demonstrate to the patient who otherwise may be quite fit or strong that they are unable to perform an apparently simple task such as drawing in their abdomen away from the pressure sensor in the prone test. It is also necessary for the patient to understand that the problem, in the transversus abdominis in particular, is one of motor control, and the type of training required can be likened to training a skill. Precision and focus is required to retrain the muscle activation, as would be needed to train any other fine skill in work or sport.

## Muscle control for pain control

The majority of patients who present for treatment of their back condition are primarily interested in obtaining relief of their back pain. Regaining muscle control and support of the injured lumbar segment will assist in relieving pain, and this is a potent 'selling point' for the programme. In addition, a considerable number of patients have been suffering recurrent and chronic pain or have gained only temporary relief from previous treatments, and are actively seeking exercise that may help them more effectively in the long term. Compliance with the exercises ceases to be an issue when patients observe that, once they can achieve activation of their deep muscles, their backs feel safer or they can control their pain.

## Introducing exercise

The picture that the clinician needs to convey to the patient is that with acute or chronic injury there is likely to be damage, for example to the disc or zygapophyseal joint. Therefore, there is loss of integrity in the passive subsystem in variable amounts. Other structures or systems must be optimized to counter this deficit in ligamentous support.

Support by the deep muscles can accommodate this deficit, and muscle control of the lumbar segment is required to protect and support the injured segment and control the pain in both the healing phase and in the long term, knowing the limited healing capacity of structures such as the disc. The irony is that the muscle system so badly needed to protect and substitute for the injured passive structures in the control of the spinal segment is also dysfunctional from the very beginning. Our research into acute, first-episode low back pain[136,139] has demonstrated that inhibition of the deep stabilizing lumbar multifidus muscle occurred virtually immediately following the onset of low back pain. The transversus abdominis has been shown to have motor control problems which can severely compromise its important contribution to lumbar spine stabilization.[146,147] Logically, the introduction of exercise strategies to reactivate and train the segmental muscle supporting system should commence as soon as possible. It is advocated that, ideally, this is in the first treatment session, regardless of whether the condition is acute or chronic. Restoration of muscle support is linked with pain control.

Clinicians often encounter patients who, once the acute pain has subsided, are not interested in further treatment or exercise. It is the responsibility of the clinician to ensure that the patient understands, if they have not already experienced it, that back pain has a high tendency for recurrence and chronicity. Local muscle support is one of their major natural defences against re-injury and pain, and training deep muscle control is a potent prevention strategy. Introducing the muscle re-education programme early in the treatment programme also obviates the need to subject the patient to additional treatments and costs which may occur with a delay in its introduction.

## Selecting the exercise strategy

In Chapter 9 various strategies were described which can be used to reactivate the deep supporting muscles. The nature of the patient's condition, often their inherent motor control abilities, their kinesthetic awareness, and the extent of their impairment are all factors that may influence which exercise strategy will be successful for the individual. In treatment, the clinician must quickly try a variety of strategies to determine which may most successfully activate the deep muscles. Precision in exercise is a key, especially with the knowledge that the transversus abdominis in its stabilizing role is operated by a separate control system from the other abdominal muscles.[152] On the basis of this evidence, accepting a compromise of a general global abdominal muscle contraction is unlikely to achieve the desired retraining of the transversus abdominis in its stabilization role.

## Repetition

With evidence of a motor-control timing deficit in the transversus abdominis, an aim of treatment is to increase the excitability of the motor neuron pool and cognitively change the motor command to return this muscle to its role of supporting the lumbopelvic region. This means that the prescription of muscle activation must focus on high repetition. The number of times a patient performs the abdominal drawing-in co-activation should be maximal and be a balance between regular opportunity and the avoidance of fatigue, which may introduce the possibility of the patient substituting incorrect muscle action. It is necessary that patients can perceive the correct muscle action and recognize fatigue so that they cease practice at that time. It is recommended that patients practise roughly on the hour, and hold the contraction while continuing a normal breathing pattern for at least 10 s. This regime also trains endurance of both the transversus abdominis and the lumbar multifidus muscles.

## Cues to practise

Unfortunately, few of us have lives that are predictable enough to exercise precisely on the hour every hour. As keen as patients may be to comply with the exercise, their attention is easily distracted from the task and they forget to practise the muscle activation, due to attention to the day's activities and work. It is therefore advantageous to discuss events during the day that may cue patients to practise, and to identify times when they are involved in activities that require little of their attention. For example, many people at work or at home answer the telephone frequently during the day. The telephone ring provides a good cue to assume an upright neutral posture and activate and hold the deep muscle co-activation. It does not matter if, once they are involved in the conversation, they relax the muscle contraction. The 10 s attention span to the exercise is usually achieved. All patients are aware of time spent sitting in traffic, sitting on buses or trains, or daily walking activities. These are ideal times for practice. Fitting exercise periods into patients', often busy, lifestyles without compromising their time is an attractive format and one that is more easily acceptable and achievable. Discuss options with the patient and, ideally, encourage them to suggest cues and times that would match their daily activities.

## Achieving the isolated contraction

In some patients it is difficult to facilitate a deep muscle contraction in relative isolation from often overactive synergists. In those cases it is easy for the clinician to become frustrated, often before the patient, and to consider the whole precision exercise strategy too difficult. Some patients do take time to learn the activation. While some patients will be able to achieve some activation in the first treatment session or over the first few days of practice, others may take several weeks. Patients have to be allowed time on their own to practise and learn the skill. Facilitation of the local muscle co-contraction is a therapeutic skill, and clinicians will improve their own skills with repetition and practice.

## Frequency of treatment

As with any skill learning, it is difficult to predict how long it will take an individual patient to learn and train the skill of activating and holding the specific deep, local muscle contraction. From the perspective of retraining the muscles, both the clinician and the patient must appreciate that the time required by an individual patient to learn the skill to activate the deep muscles will be variable and be in response to several factors. These could include patients' inherent motor skills, the extent of the motor control deficit associated with their back problem, influences of pain and reflex inhibition and, indeed, the teaching and facilitation skills of the clinician. Individuals with good coordination and body awareness will quickly learn the skill and become proficient in a relatively short period of time, while others will need a longer period of dedicated practice to achieve the same level. The experienced and skilled clinician will gain a reasonable estimate of patients' potential efficiency at the time of the initial assessment, based on their response to various facilitation strategies. The time can vary from several days to several weeks.

The frequency of treatment sessions relates to patients' ability to learn the muscle actions. In the initial stages of management of either acute or chronic back pain patients, the number of sessions should be sufficient to ensure that the patient is achieving and practising the correct muscle actions. Once this has been achieved, sessions should be spaced appropriately to allow time for retraining. Facilitation and retraining should, whenever possible, be commenced in the first treatment session along with treatments for other systems which are directed towards relief of pain and restoration of spinal movement. During management of the painful stage, this permits regular teaching and reassessment. When exercise becomes the focus of management it is usually most efficient, both in terms of exercise effect and cost, to space treatment sessions. This applies both to the subacute patient and the patient with persistent pain who primarily seeks treatment to prevent recurrence. Patients need to be given the chance to practise to achieve the muscle activation, before there can be rational, safe and logical progression through the stages of the programme.

## Training in functional positions

Training the activation of the deep, local muscles in functional positions such as standing and sitting serves several purposes. Repetition is a key to successful retraining when the aim is to increase the excitability of the motor neuron pool and cognitively change a motor command to counter a dysfunction in the motor control of a muscle. While the supine lying or side lying positions may be used for initial teaching and facilitation of transversus abdominis and multifidus activation, they are not convenient positions for practice during the day on a regular basis. For this reason, the patient is taught activation strategies in standing or sitting as soon as possible, which they can easily and conveniently incorporate frequently into their daily routine. In addition, activation of this deep muscle corset will provide support and control to the lumbar segments during everyday activities such as sitting, standing, bending and walking. Patient observations such as 'my back feels safer' and 'I can control my pain' by practising and using the abdominal drawing-in action in function is a powerful incentive for compliance.

## Training the outer muscle unit

Training the outer muscle unit can be safely commenced once control of the inner muscle unit, and hence control at the lumbar segmental level, has been achieved. To delay the introduction of this more conventional type of exercise until the patient can successfully activate and hold the deep muscle co-activation is often a source of frustration to the clinician and patient alike. However, there is always the temptation to introduce these exercises too early, and this can do more harm than good. General exercise with load may render an uncontrolled segment vulnerable to strain. Furthermore, the nature of the motor-control dysfunction in the transversus abdominis indicates that, if the rehabilitation approach focuses on general exercises such as sit-ups alone, there is a risk that the muscle will act with the torque producers and not resume its stabilization function.

Training of the outer muscle unit and its interaction with the deep muscles is an important component of stabilization training, but exercise must be undertaken as precisely and carefully as when training the inner muscle unit. Initial exercise strategies are of a low-load nature. They should be performed slowly and carefully so that maintenance of control of a neutral spine position can be achieved. When leg load is used to challenge the trunk muscle co-activation, the patient's ability to hold and control a stable position of the lumbopelvic region can be monitored objectively using the pressure biofeedback unit. This feedback about the ability to control the lumbopelvic posture soon convinces the clinician and patient of the need to begin exercise with low load when muscle control is the key element of training.

Progression of the programme challenges the muscle system through added load and more unstable positions. Caution must be applied in the rate of progression. Clinicians and patients must resist the temptation to progress too quickly to levels that the patient is unable to control. Such exercise becomes counterproductive to the aim of the programme, i.e. to enhance muscle stabilization capacity. If this capacity is exceeded by the exercise, the patient will adopt inappropriate strategies to cope with the task, which may not only be ineffectual but may also risk adverse strain on the lumbar motion segment. The degree of flattening of the abdomen and lumbopelvic position should always be monitored. The extent of the loads and speeds incorporated into the exercise programme should match the functional and recreational demands of the patient and will therefore vary between different patients.

## Reassessment of the inner muscle unit

It is necessary at all stages of the exercise programme to ensure that the patient maintains the ability to activate and hold the deep muscle co-activation. For this reason, it is recommended that the quantifiable prone test of the abdominal drawing-in action is done regularly throughout the entire treatment period. Furthermore, at this stage of our knowledge, it is recommended that the patient continually self-check the action on a regular basis, even when their pain has subsided and they have been discharged from formal treatment. In some patients, once the action has been retrained, they retain the skill, whereas in others the skill needs to be refreshed at regular intervals. A weekly self-check after discharge is often prescribed. If the patient considers that their ability has decreased or they develop 'that feel' of vulnerability in their backs, then a concentrated period of practice is in order. Maintaining the function of the inner muscle unit affords protection to the lumbar segments in the quest for prevention of re-injury and chronic and recurrent back pain.

# Future directions

One of the exciting outcomes of the continual interaction between scientific and clinical development is the potential for refinement of the clinical approach on the basis of scientific evidence and the development of scientific ideas on the basis of clinical findings. This must result in better health care delivery and eventually to the control and prevention of the debilitating condition of low back pain.

# 12

# Future directions in research and clinical practice

The stringent analyses of the effectiveness of many current conservative treatment methods for low back pain through the research technique of meta-analysis have not produced strong evidence in favour of a particular method or methods.[190,191,193,341] They have also produced evidence that certain treatments should be abandoned. While reasons may be offered for the seeming lack of performance of some of the treatment approaches, the message must come through that there needs to be a constant search for new knowledge about the musculoskeletal dysfunction in low back pain, and new evidence-based directions in treatment developed to solve this enigmatic problem.

This book has presented the scientific argument and clinical reasoning that was involved in the development of a completely new exercise approach for the management of low back pain. The new method aims to achieve pain control and to address the recurrence of back pain by selectively exercising specific muscles from a synergistic group in order to enhance their unique features of supporting and protecting from injury the spinal segment and lumbopelvic area. In the future, the method may direct measures to prevent the first occurrence of low back pain.

The new concept involves exercises using only relatively low activity levels in the muscles. More emphasis is placed on a motor skill which has to be relearned, practised and then gradually incorporated back into functional movement. These specific muscle contractions involve a group of muscles close to the spine which, we believe, act as a single unit to provide support to the lumbopelvic region, seemingly operating independently of the muscles which move or brace the trunk in functional tasks. This division in muscle system function is logical and efficient for bodily function. The global system of larger muscles is responsible for responding to the external environment, to minimize the resulting force and damaging load on the lumbopelvic region. The system of deep muscles lying close to the spine is specialized for joint protection at a local level. Most importantly, it has been argued that it is the muscles in this latter system which are most affected in the low back pain patient, and it is impairment in the function of this system which is linked to the high recurrence rate seen in this condition.

Interestingly, a similar approach to the treatment of a musculoskeletal condition has also been developed for the neck, shoulder, hip and knee regions. Again, specific muscles linked to joint support rather than joint movement seem to be most affected by injury to the region, and these muscles are trained separately and independently as the first step in the rehabilitation process.

## ASSESSING THE LOCAL STABILIZING MUSCLES OF THE SPINE

It is widely acknowledged that outcome measures which reflect impairments in the muscle system are essential to proving the efficacy of the various types of therapeutic exercise in treating back pain. In this age of technological advancement, highly accurate, sophisticated and repeatable measurement techniques have been developed for assessing the strength and endurance of most movements of the body, even in three dimensions. However, these measures have not raised the question of or exposed the presence of deep local muscle dysfunction in low back pain, nor do they provide the answers to how the impairments in deep muscles can be assessed. The development of these assessments has been made more difficult due to the location of the target muscles deep in the body and close to the

spine. The assessments may be difficult to comprehend initially, as these muscles cannot be seen from the surface of the body and their contractions do not result in movement of the trunk or limbs as is usually required for measurements of skeletal muscle function.

Quantification is gradually being achieved, with scientists working closely with those who treat back pain patients. While invasive measures have been described using fine-wire electromyography (EMG), there is a great need for valid non-invasive measures that have wider application. A combined measure using ultrasound imaging, surface EMG and pressure recordings is currently being developed. Preliminary data using the interrelationship between these three modalities are promising, but other methods should be investigated. In the management of the back pain patient, new non-invasive assessments may provide detailed information about the degree of motor control deficit, and hence direct the type and specificity of therapeutic exercise required to achieve a good long-term result for the individual patient.

It is acknowledged that we have not specifically assessed several muscles of the local system, such as the medial fibres of quadratus lumborum, the lumbar longissimus and iliocostalis, for specific dysfunction in relation to segmental stabilization in the back pain patient. This promises to be an interesting area for future research.

## THE TREATMENT TECHNIQUE

Treatment of deep muscle impairment, as we have described, does not involve the use of a standard approach. The facilitation techniques necessary to achieve the isolated contraction of the deep muscles without the contraction of the global muscles can vary for each patient. Assessment of the individual patient followed by clinical problem-solving of their particular pattern of muscle performance holds the key to choosing successful treatment techniques. It is fair to say that the treatment procedures described in this book do demand high levels of clinical skill and practice. These high levels of clinical skill are necessary to prevent the negative consequences of allowing the patient to perform poor patterns, which can be reinforced in their home exercises and result in no improvement or even a worsening of their condition. Another challenge for the clinician is to help motivate the patient to perform these precise exercise routines as frequently as possible during the day. It is skill retraining that requires precision and repetition. The clinician's skill in 'selling' the concept of this different form of exercise will impact on their personal success in using the method. Having an evidence base for the exercises makes this task easier.

One question that is often asked of us is what level of precision is required to gain the most effective results in the minimum of time? Our current opinion is that it is necessary to reach a high level of precision of the skill, i.e. where negligible contribution of global muscles occurs with the deep, local muscle cocontraction. This is based on experience in our back pain clinic, where real-time ultrasound is available to help with assessment and facilitation. The future may see this question of the level of precision required in training the motor skill answered quite quickly. This is possible with the increasing knowledge available on methods of optimally learning a new motor skill, as well as the possibilities of new research directed towards the specific problems in back pain patients.

Besides the area of relearning a motor skill, there are many directions for future research into optimal treatment methods. Some include finding the ways in which the contraction of specific pelvic floor muscles as well as the diaphragm can help achieve the isolated contractions of the transversus abdominis and lumbar multifidus for the re-education process. The use of real-time ultrasound as a biofeedback tool in the re-learning phase of rehabilitation needs specific investigation to ensure its efficacy and its safety when used repetitively in treatment programmes rather than its more usual use in medical diagnosis. Another question that relates to patients with overactive global muscles, is what methods will optimally help to decrease the activity of muscles such as the obliquus

externus abdominis or internus during retraining of the deep muscle action. The use of different breathing patterns, pelvic belts, posturing on large gym balls, and inhibitory muscle stroking are some options yet to be investigated.

## MECHANISMS

The mechanisms of action of the specific exercise programme are not clear at present, but they are likely to include both biomechanical and physiological factors. The role of the lumbar multifidus in providing segmental support has been studied closely (see Ch. 3) and there is a growing understanding of how the transversus abdominis can contribute to spinal segmental control (see Ch. 4). The deep muscles, transversus abdominis and lumbar multifidus, are closely linked to the fascias, which encircle the lumbar spine and pelvis. In a conceptual model, as their action causes a tightening of the fascias, these deep muscles could be seen as being part of a dynamic active fascial system of support for the lumbar and pelvic joints. Biomechanical models need to be constructed to demonstrate that active support of the intervertebral segments and sacro-iliac joints can be achieved by the deep myofascial system independently of the actions of the muscles whose role it is to move and control the displacements of the whole trunk and limbs.

Neurophysiological studies are required to extend our knowledge of the nervous system in order to explain the mechanisms involved in spinal and postural support and the changes that occur when pathology is involved. Several factors require investigation: the challenge for the central nervous system to integrate and coordinate the respiratory and postural functions of the diaphragm; the mechanisms of muscle synergies in spinal support; clarification of the specific control of the local group of fibres of the lumbar multifidus; the responses of the trunk muscles to other types of perturbation; the bilateral co-activation of the transversus abdominis; and the mechanism of the delayed postural activation of the trunk muscles. The possible physiological and biochemical effects in the effector organs, muscles and fascias also need to be studied.

There are likely to be other mechanisms that require investigation. These include the likelihood of contraction of the deep muscles increasing the circulation to the spinal structures and assisting the healing of injured tissue. It is possible that the contraction could provide very specific sensory input, which could help with the modulation of pain at various levels in the central nervous system. Future basic science research is needed to prove or disprove these possible mechanisms.

This biomechanical, physiological and biochemical research is needed to explain the essence of active control of segmental movement. Some of these studies would need to continue hand in hand with clinical research to find the reason why training of the deep myofascial systems could be producing clinical effects of controlling pain and persistent episodes of low back pain.

## WHO BENEFITS FROM THERAPEUTIC EXERCISE?

There are many types of therapeutic exercise recommended for the back pain patient, ranging from aggressive strength training, to general stability programmes, to exercises to enhance cardiovascular fitness. Many of these programmes result in functional benefits for patients, increasing their activity level and giving them a feeling of well-being. The uniqueness of the specific exercises described in this book is that they target pain relief directly, as well as the control of persistent episodes of low back pain.

We believe that all patients who suffer low back pain require this specific exercise training and this is based on our experience of the seemingly universal reaction in the deep muscles to back injury and pain.[136,146,257,259] This does not dismiss the benefits of or the need for other types of exercise. Notably, it does not deny the possibility that other methods and techniques of exercise currently in use could result in successful retraining of the deep muscle supporting function. The provision of valid non-invasive

measures of deep muscle function will allow the effect of such programmes to be investigated. What we do contend is that retraining of the deep muscles needs to become an integral part of rehabilitation of low back pain patients, such retraining providing a foundation for the safe performance of more general exercise programmes directed at general stability, strength or cardiovascular fitness. There is a group of patients whom we do believe should withdraw from other types of exercise training to receive only specific and precise deep muscle training until the deep muscle function is restored. These are the patients who are suffering quite debilitating persistent or recurrent problems, for often they have quite significant motor control problems which can be perpetuated by general exercise and which in turn hinder any hope of successful re-education of deep muscle supporting function.

The specific exercises used to target the deep muscles potentially have many other benefits that need to be addressed in future research. The provision of increased 'core' stability may result in better coordination and use of the more distal pelvic and limb muscles, and enhance the general muscle performance of the individual. In addition, athletic trainers, as well as healthcare practitioners, could benefit from studying the effects of improving core stability on their current strength training regimes.

Our increased understanding of the supporting function of the deep muscles for the back and the interrelationship of muscle groups to provide this support is relevant to the treatment of other conditions. For example, the treatment of muscles of the pelvic floor for conditions such as stress incontinence and constipation[297] is being refined as the close associations between these pelvic floor muscles and the deep muscles supporting the back are being revealed. The knowledge of the relationships between specific muscles of the abdominal wall and specific muscles of the pelvic floor offer very real possibilities for more effective treatments of conditions involving the rehabilitation of the muscles of the pelvic floor.

The link between the deep trunk muscles, the

diaphragm and breathing patterns offers another area of unexplained questions in muscle function and re-education alternatives. Could it be that training deep muscle function in the trunk could be used to influence respiratory patterns? Does this have any potential benefit for the treatment of chest conditions, where efficient functioning of the diaphragm is required? These are new research questions, the practical significance of which is currently under investigation.

Future research into the deep muscles of the trunk abounds with possibilities for those interested in the treatment and prevention of back pain, and knowledge in this area should escalate. The combination of new knowledge about the impairments in the muscle system linked to low back pain, new technologies and fresh directions of thinking for therapeutic exercise places physical therapy in a good position to meet the challenges of providing effective and efficient evidence-based practices.

# References

1. Abe T, Kusuhara N, Yoshimura N, Tomita T, Easton P A 1996 Differential respiratory activity of four abdominal muscles in humans. Journal of Applied Physiology 80:1379–1389

2. Abernethy B, Kippers V, Mackinnon L T, Neal R J, Hanrahan S 1996 The biophysical foundations of human movement. Macmillan, Melbourne

3. Abumi K, Panjabi M M, Kramer K M, Duranceau J, Oxland T, Crisco J J 1990 Biomechanical evaluation of lumbar spinal stability after graded facetectomies. Spine 15:1142–1147

4. Adams M A 1991 Letter to the editor. Spine 16:483

5. Agostoni E, Sant'Ambrogio G 1970 The diaphragm. In: Campbell E J M, Agostoni E, Newsom–Davis J (eds) The respiratory muscles: mechanisms and neural control. Lloyd-Luke, London, pp 145–160

6. Alaranta H, Tallroth K, Soukka A, Heliovaara M 1993 Fat content of lumbar extensor muscles and low back disability: a radiographic and clinical comparison. Journal of Spinal Disorders 6:137–140

7. Alexander C J 1972 In-vivo estimation of vein-wall tension and hoop stress. The Medical Journal of Australia 1:311–313

8. Allison G T, Kendle K, Roll S, Schipelius J, Scott Q, Panizza J A 1997 The role of the diaphragm during abdominal hollowing exercises. Australian Journal of Physiotherapy 44(2): 95–102

9. Allum J H J, Honegger F, Platz C R 1989 The role of stretch and vestibulospinal reflexes in the generation of human equilibrating reactions. Afferent control of posture and locomotion. In: Allum J H J, Hulliger M (eds) Progress in brain research. Elsevier, Amsterdam, pp 399–409

10. Amonoo-Kuofi H S 1983 The density of muscle spindles in the medial, intermediate and lateral columns of human intrinsic post-vertebral muscles. Journal of Anatomy 136:509–519

11. Andersson E, Ma Z, Nilsson J, Thorstensson A 1989 Abdominal and hip flexor muscle involvement in various training exercises. In: Proceedings from the XII International Congress of Biomechanics, Los Angeles, pp 254–255

12. Andersson E A, Oddsson L I E, Grundstrom O M, Nilsson J, Thorstensson A 1996 EMG activities of the quadratus lumborum and erector spinae muscles during flexion–relaxation and other motor tasks. Clinical Biomechanics 11:392–400

13. Andersson G, Bogduk N, DeLuca C et al 1989 Muscle. In: Frymoyer J W, Gordon S L (eds) New perspectives on low back pain. American Academy of Orthopaedic Surgeons, Illinois ch 7, pp 291–230

14. Anderson R, Meeker W, Wirick B, Mootz R, Kirk D, Adams A 1992 A meta-analysis of clinical trials of spinal manipulation. Journal of Manipulative and Physiological Therapeutics 14:181–194

15. Angel R W 1974 Electromyography during voluntary movement: the two-burst pattern. Electroencephalography and Clinical Neurophysiology 36:493–498

16. Appell H J 1990 Muscular atrophy following immobilisation: a review. Sports Medicine 10:42–58

17. Aruin A S, Latash M L 1995 Directional specificity of postural muscles in feed-forward postural reactions during fast voluntary arm movements. Experimental Brain Research 103:323–332

18. Ashton-Miller J A, Schultz A B 1991 Spine instability and segmental hypermobility biomechanics: a call for the definition and standard use of terms. Seminars of Spine Surgery 3:136–148

19. Askar O M 1977 Surgical anatomy of the aponeurotic expansions of the anterior abdominal wall. Annals of the Royal College of Surgeons of England 59:313–321

20. Asmussen E, Klausen K 1962 Form and function of the erect human spine. Clinical Orthopaedics and Related Research 25:55–63

21. Aspden R M 1987 Intra-abdominal pressure and its role in spinal mechanics. Clinical Biomechanics 2:168–174

22. Aspden R M 1989 The spine as an arch: a new mathematical model. Spine 14:266–274

23. Aspden R M 1992 Review of the functional anatomy of the spinal ligaments and the lumbar erector spinae muscles. Clinical Anatomy 5:372–387

24. Bagnall K M, Ford D M, McFadden K D, Greenhill B J, Raso V J 1984 The histochemical composition of human vertebral muscle. Spine 9:470–473

25. Baratta R, Solomonow M, Zhou B H, Letson D, Chuinard R, D'Ambrosia E 1988 Muscular activation. The role of the antagonist musculature in maintaining knee stability. The American Journal of Sports Medicine 16:113–122

26. Bartelink D L 1957 The role of intra-abdominal pressure in relieving the pressure on the lumbar vertebral discs. Journal of Bone and Joint Surgery 39B:718–725

27. Basmajian J V, DeLuca C J 1985 Muscles alive – their functions revealed by electromyography, 5th edn. Williams & Wilkins, Baltimore

28. Baxendale R H, Ferrell W R, Wood L 1987 The effect of mechanical stimulation of knee joint afferents on quadriceps motor unit activity in the decerebrate cat. Brain Research 415:353–356

29. Bearn J G 1961 The significance of the activity of the abdominal muscles in weight lifting. Acta Anatomica 45:83–89

30. Beckerman H, Bouter L M, van de Heijden G J, DeBie R A, Koes B W 1993 Efficacy of physiotherapy for musculoskeletal disorders: What can we learn from research? British Journal of General Practice 43:73–77

31. Bednar H H 1986 Pressure vessel design handbook. Krieger, Malabar, FL

32. Belen'kii V, Gurfinkel V S, Paltsev Y 1967 Elements of control of voluntary movements. Biofizika 12:135–141

33. Bergmark A 1989 Stability of the lumbar spine. A study in mechanical engineering. Acta Orthopaedica Scandinavica 230(suppl):20–24

34. Biedermann H J, Shanks G L, Forrest W J, Inglis J 1991 Power spectrum analysis of electromyographic activity: discriminators in the differential assessment of patients with chronic low back pain. Spine 16:1179–1185

35. Blasier R B, Carpenter J E, Huston L J 1994 Shoulder proprioception: effect on joint laxity, joint position and direction. Orthopaedic Review 23:45–50

36. Boden S D, Weisel S W 1990 Lumbosacral segmental motion in normal individuals. Have we been measuring instability properly? Spine 15:571–576

37. Bogduk N 1997 Clinical anatomy of the lumbar spine and sacrum, 3rd edn. Churchill Livingstone, Edinburgh

38. Bogduk N, Macintosh J E 1984 The applied anatomy of the thoracolumbar fascia. Spine 9:164–170

39. Bogduk N, Macintosh J E, Pearcy M J 1992 A universal model of the lumbar back muscles in the upright position. Spine 17:897–913

40. Bogduk N, Pearcy M, Hadfield G 1992 Anatomy and biomechanics of the psoas major. Clinical Biomechanics 7:109–119

41. Bogduk N, Wilson A S, Tynan W 1982 The lumbar dorsal rami. Journal of Anatomy 134:383–397

42. Bouisset S, Zattara M 1981 A sequence of postural adjustments precedes voluntary movement. Neuroscience Letters 22:263–270

43. Bradford D S, Cooper KM, Omega T R 1983 Chymopapin, chemonucleosis and nucleus pulposus regeneration. Journal of Bone and Joint Surgery 65A:1220–1231

44. Bullock-Saxton J E 1994 Local sensation and altered hip muscle function following severe ankle sprain. Physical Therapy 74:17–31

45. Burke R E, Edgerton V R 1975 Unit properties and selective involvement in movement. Exercise and Sports Science Reviews 3:31–81

46. Byl N N, Sinnott P L 1991 Variations in balance and body sway in middle-aged adults: subjects with healthy backs compared with subjects with low back dysfunction. Spine 16:325–330

47. Campbell E J M 1952 An electromyographic study of the role of the abdominal muscles in breathing. Journal of Physiology 117:222–233

48. Campbell E J M, Green J H 1955 The behaviour of the abdominal muscles and the intra-abdominal pressure during quiet breathing and increased pulmonary ventilation. Journal of Physiology 127:423–426

49. Carman D J, Blanton P L, Biggs N L 1972 Electromyographic study of the antero-lateral abdominal musculature using indwelling electrodes. American Journal of Physical Medicine 15:113–129

50. Carolan B, Catarelli E 1992 Adaptations in coactivation after isometric resistance training. Journal of Applied Physiology 73:911–917

51. Cassisi J E, Robinson M E, O'Connor P, MacMillan M 1993 Trunk strength and lumbar paraspinal muscle activity during isometric exercise in chronic low back pain patients and controls. Spine 18:245–251

52. Charman R A 1997 Motor learning. In: Trew M, Everett T (eds) Human movement, 3rd edn. Churchill Livingstone, Edinburgh, ch 5, pp 87–104

53. Cholewicki J, McGill S 1992 Lumbar posterior ligament involvement during extremely heavy lifts estimated from fluoroscopic measurement. Journal of Biomechanics 25:17–28

54. Cholewicki J, McGill S M 1996 Mechanical stability of the in vivo lumbar spine: implications for injury and low back pain. Clinical Biomechanics 11:1–15

55. Cholewicki J, McGill S M, Norman R W 1991 Lumbar spine loads during the lifting of extremely heavy weights. Medicine and Science in Sports and Exercise 23:1179–1186

56. Cholewicki J, Panjabi M M, Khachatryan A 1997 Stabilizing function of trunk flexor–extensor muscles around a neutral spine posture. Spine 22:2207–2212

57. Conley M S, Meyer R A, Bloomberg J J, Feeback D L, Dudley G A 1995 Noninvasive analysis of human neck muscle function. Spine 20:2505–2512

58. Cooper R G, Clair Forbes W S T, Jayson M I V 1992 Radiographic demonstration of paraspinal muscle wasting in patients with chronic low back pain. British Journal of Rheumatology 31:389–394

59. Cordo P J, Nashner, L M 1982 Properties of postural adjustments associated with rapid arm movements. Journal of Neurophysiology 47:287–308

60. Craig A D, Heppelmann B, Schaible H G 1988 The projection of the medial and posterior articular nerves of the cat's knee to the spinal cord. Journal of Comparative Neurology 276:279–288

61. Cram J R, Steger J C 1983 EMG scanning in the diagnosis of chronic pain. Biofeedback and Self Regulation 8:229–241

62. Cresswell A G 1993 Responses of intra-abdominal pressure and abdominal muscle activity during dynamic trunk loading in man. European Journal of Applied Physiology 66:315–320

63. Cresswell A G, Blake P L, Thorstensson A 1993 The effect of an abdominal muscle training program on the intra-abdominal pressure. Sandinavian Journal of Rehabilitation Medicine 26:79–86

64. Cresswell A G, Grundstrom A, Thorstensson A 1992 Observations on intra-abdominal pressure and patterns of abdominal intra-muscular activity in man. Acta Physiologica Scandinavica 144:409–418

65. Cresswell A G, Oddsson L, Thorstensson A 1994 The influence of sudden perturbations on trunk muscle activity and intra-abdominal pressure while standing. Experimental Brain Research 98:336–341

66. Cresswell A G, Thorstensson A 1989 The role of the abdominal musculature in the elevation of the intra-abdominal pressure during specific tasks. Ergonomics 32:1237–1246

67. Cresswell A G, Thorstensson A 1994 Change in intra-abdominal pressure, trunk muscle activation and force during isokinetic lifting and lowering. European Journal of Applied Physiology 68:315–321

68. Crisco J J, Panjabi M M 1991 The intersegmental and multisegmental muscles of the spine: a biomechanical model comparing lateral stabilising potential. Spine 7:793–799

69. Crisco J J, Panjabi M M, Yamamoto I, Oxland T R 1992 Euler stability of the human ligamentous lumbar spine. Clinical Biomechanics 7:27–32

70. Culham L C, Peat M 1993 Functional anatomy of the shoulder complex. Journal of Orthopaedic and Sports Physical Therapy 18:342–350

71. Daggfeldt K, Thorstensson A 1991 The role of intra-abdominal pressure in spinal unloading. Journal of Biomechanics 30:1149–1155

72. Damiano D L 1993 Reviewing muscle co-contraction: is it a developmental, pathological or motor control issue? Physical and Occupational Therapy in Paediatrics 12:3–20

73. David G C 1985 Intra-abdominal pressure measurements and load capabilities for females. Ergonomics 28:345–358

74. Davis P R 1956 Variations of intra-abdominal pressure during weight lifting in various postures. Journal of Anatomy 90:601

75. Davis P R 1959 Posture of the trunk during the lifting of weights. British Medical Journal 1:87–89

76. Davis P R 1981 The use of intra-abdominal pressure in evaluating stresses on the lumbar spine. Spine 6:90–92

77. Davis, P R, Troup J D G 1964 Pressures in the trunk cavity when pulling, pushing and lifting. Ergonomics 7:465–474

78. DeAndre J R, Grant C, Dixon A S J 1965 Joint distension and reflex muscle inhibition in the knee. Journal of Bone and Joint Surgery 47A:313–322

79. Delhez, L 1968 Motor activity of the respiratory system. Poumon et Le Coeur 24:845–888

80. DeSerres S J, Milner T E 1991 Wrist muscle activation patterns and stiffness associated with stable and unstable mechnical loads. Experimental Brain Research 86:451–458

81. DeTroyer A 1983 Mechanical role of the abdominal muscles in relation to posture. Respiration Physiology 53:341–353

82. DeTroyer A, Estenne M 1988 Functional anatomy of the respiratory muscles. In: Belman M J (ed) Respiratory muscles: function in health and disease. W B Saunders, Philadelphia, vol 9, pp 175–195

83. DeTroyer A, Estenne M, Ninane V, VanGansbeke D, Gorini M 1990 Transversus abdominis muscle function in humans. Journal of Applied Physiology 68:1010–1016

84. Dolce J J, Raczynski J M 1985 Neuromuscular activity and electromyography in painful backs: physiological and biomechanical models in assessment and treatment. Psychological Bulletin 97:502–520

85. Donisch E W, Basmajian J V 1972 Electromyography of deep back muscles in man. American Journal of Anatomy 133:15–36

86. Eccles R M, Lundberg A 1959 Synaptic actions in motoneurones by afferents which may evoke the flexion reflex. Archives Italiennes de Biologie 97:199–221

87. Ecleshymer A C, Schoemaker D M 1970 A cross-sectional anatomy. Butterworths, London

88. Edstrom L 1970 Selective atrophy of red muscles in the quadriceps in long standing knee joint dysfunction: injuries to the anterior cruciate ligament. Journal of the Neurological Sciences 11:551–558

89. Ekholm J, Eklund G, Skoglund S 1960 On reflex effects from knee joint of cats. Acta Physiologica Scandinavica 50:167–174

90. Fairbank J C T, O'Brien J P, Davis P R 1980 Intra-abdominal pressure rise during weight lifting as an objective measure of low-back pain. Spine 5:179–184

91. Farfan H F 1973 Mechanical disorders of the low back. Lea & Febiger, Philadelphia

92. Farfan H F 1975 Muscular mechanism of the lumbar spine and the position of power and efficiency. Orthopedic Clinics of North America 6:135–145

93. Farfan H F, Gracovetsky S, Helleur C 1983 The role of mathematical models in the assessment of tasks in the workplace. In: Winter D A, Norman R W, Wells P R, Hayes C, Patza A (eds) Biomechanics IX-B Human Kinetics, Champaign, IL, pp 38–43

94. Fidler M W, Jowett R L, Troup J D G 1975 Myosin ATPase activity in multifidus muscle from cases of lumbar spinal derangement. Journal of Bone and Joint Surgery 57B:220–227

95. Fitts R H, Brimmer C J 1985 Recovery in skeletal muscle contractile function after prolonged hindlimb immobilization. Journal of Applied Physiology 59:916–923

96. Floyd W F, Silver P H S 1950 Electromyographic study of patterns of activity of the anterior abdominal wall muscles in man. Journal of Anatomy 84:132–145

97. Floyd W F, Silver P H S 1951 Function of erector spinae in flexion of the trunk. Lancet 20:133–134

98. Ford D, Bagnall K M, McFadden H D, Greenhill B, Raso J 1983 Analysis of vertebral muscle obtained during surgery for correction of a lumbar disc disorder. Acta Anatomica 116:152–157

99. Fregosi R F, Hwang J-C, Bartlett D, StJohn W M 1992 Activity of abdominal muscle motoneurons during hypercapnia. Respiration Physiology 89:179–194

100. Friedli W G, Hallet M, Simon S R 1984 Postural adjustments associated with rapid voluntary arm movements 1. Electromyographic data. Journal of Neurology, Neurosurgery and Psychiatry 47:611–622

101. Friedman P, Eisen G 1980 The Pilates method of physical and mental condition. Doubleday, New York

102. Frymoyer J W, Pope M H 1991 Segmental instability. Seminars of Spine Surgery 3:109–118

103. Frymoyer J W, Pope M H, Wilder D G 1990 Segmental instability. In: Weinstein J N, Wiesel S (eds) The lumbar spine. W B Saunders, Philadelphia, pp 612–636

104. Fukushima H, Hinoki M 1985 Role of the cervical and lumbar proprioceptors during stepping: an electromyographic study of the muscular activities of the lower limbs. Acta Otolaryngologica (Stockholm) 419 (suppl):91–105

105. Gardner E 1950 Reflex muscular responses to stimulation of articular nerves in the cat. American Journal of Physiology 161:133–141

106. Gardner-Morse M, Stokes I A F, Lauble J P 1995 Role of the muscles in lumbar spine stability in maximum extension efforts. Journal of Orthopaedic Research 13:802–808

107. Gaskell D V, Webber B A 1980 The Brompton Hospital guide to chest physiotherapy. Blackwell Scientific, Oxford

108. Gertzbein S D, Seligman J, Holtby R et al 1985 Centrode patterns and segmental instability in degenerative disc disease. Spine 10:257–261

109. Goel V K, Gilbertson L G 1995 Applications of the finite element method to thoracolumbar spinal research – past, present and future. Spine 20:1719–1727

110. Goel V K, Kong W, Han J S, Weinstein D O, Gilbertson L G 1993 A combined finite element and optimization of lumbar spine mechanics with and without muscles. Spine 18:1531–1541

111. Goff B 1972 The application of recent advances in neurophysiology to Miss M Rood's concept of neuromuscular facilitation. Physiotherapy 58:409–415

112. Goldman J M, Lehr R P, Millar A B, Silver J R 1987 An electromyographic study of the abdominal muscles during postural and respiratory manoeuvres. Journal of Neurology, Neurosurgery and Psychiatry 50:866–869

113. Gottschalk F, Kourosh S, Leveau B 1989 The functional anatomy of tensor fascia latae and gluteus medius and minimus. Journal of Anatomy 166:179–189

114. Grabiner M D, Koh T J, Ghazawi A E 1992 Decoupling of bilateral excitation in subjects with low back pain. Spine 17:1219–1223

115. Gracovetsky S 1986 Function of the spine. Journal of Biomedical Engineering 8:217–223

116. Gracovetsky S, Farfan H, Helleur C 1985 The abdominal mechanism. Spine 10:317–324

117. Gracovetsky S, Farfan H F, Lamy C 1977 A mathematical model of the lumbar spine using an optimised system to control muscles and ligaments. Orthopedic Clinics of North America 8:135–153

118. Gracovetsky S, Farfan H F, Lamy C 1981 The mechanism of the lumbar spine. Spine 6:249–262

119. Grew N D 1980 Intraabdominal pressure response to loads applied to the torso in normal subjects. Spine 5:149–154

120. Grigg P, Harrigan E P, Fogarty K E 1978 Segmental reflexes mediated by joint afferent neurons in cat knee. Journal of Neurophysiology 41:9–14

121. Grillner S, Nilsson J, Thorstensson A 1978 Intraabdominal pressure changes during natural movements in man. Acta Physiologica Scandinavica 103:275–283

122. Guyton A C 1981 Textbook of medical physiology, 6th edn. W B Saunders, Philadelphia

123. Häggmark T, Jansson E, Eriksson E 1981 Fibre type area and metabolic potential of the thigh muscle in man after knee surgery and immobilisation. International Journal of Sports Medicine 2:2–17

124. Hamilton C, Richardson C 1995 Towards the development of a clinical test of local muscle dysfunction in the lumbar spine. In: Proceedings of the 9th Biennial Conference of the Manipulative Physiotherapists Association of Australia, Brisbane. MPAA, Melbourne, pp 54–56

125. Harman E A, Frykman P N, Clagett E R, Kraemer W J 1988 Intra-abdominal and intra-thoracic pressures during lifting and jumping. Medicine and Science in Sports and Exercise 20:195–201

126. Hayward L, Breitbach D, Rymer W Z 1988 Increased inhibitory effects on close synergists during muscle fatigue in decerebrate cat. Brain Research 440:199–203

127. He X, Proske V, Schaible H G, Schmidt R F 1988 Acute inflammation of the knee joint in the cat alters responses of flexor motoneurones to leg movements. Journal of Neurophysiology 59:326–340

128. Hebert L J, Serres S J, Arsenault A B 1991 Cocontraction of the elbow muscles during combined tasks of pronation–flexion and supination–flexion. Electromyography and Clinical Neurophysiology 31:483–488

129. Hemborg B, Moritz U, Hamberg J, Lowing H, Akesson I 1983 Intra-abdominal pressure and trunk muscle activity during lifting – effect of abdominal training in healthy subjects. Scandinavian Journal of Rehabilitation Medicine 15:183–196

130. Hemborg B, Moritz U, Löwing H 1985 Intra-abdominal pressure and trunk muscle activity during lifting. IV. The causal factors of the intra-abdominal pressure rise. Scandinavian Journal of Rehabilitation Medicine 17:25–38

131. Henke K G, Sharratt M, Pegelow D, Dempsey J A 1988 Regulation of end-expiratory lung volume during exercise. Journal of Applied Physiology 64:135–146

132. Hermann R, Mixon J, Fisher A, Maulussi R, Stuyck J 1985 Idiopathic scoliosis and the central nervous system: A motor control problem. Spine 10:1–14

133. Hides J A 1996 Multifidus muscle recovery in acute low back patients. PhD thesis, Department of Physiotherapy, The University of Queensland

134. Hides J A, Richardson C A, Jull G A 1995 Magnetic resonance imaging and ultrasonography of the lumbar multifidus muscle: Comparison of two different modalities. Spine 20:54–58

135. Hides J A, Richardson C A, Jull G A, Davies S E 1996 Ultrasound imaging in rehabilitation. Australian Journal of Physiotherapy 41:187–193

136. Hides J A, Richardson C A, Jull G A 1996 Multifidus muscle recovery is not automatic following resolution of acute first episode low back pain. Spine 21:2763–2769

137. Hides J A, Richardson C A, Jull G A 1996 Multifidus muscle rehabilitation decreases recurrence of symptoms following first episode low back pain. In: Proceedings of the National Congress of the Australian Physiotherapy Association, Brisbane

138. Hides J A, Jull G A, Richardson C A, Hodges P W 1997 Lokale Gelenkstabilisation: Spezifische Befunderhebung und Übungen bei lumbalen Ruckenschmerzen. Manuelle Therapie 1:8–15

139. Hides J A, Stokes M J, Saide M, Jull G A, Cooper D H 1994 Evidence of lumbar multifidus muscle wasting ipsilateral to symptoms in patients with acute/subacute low back pain. Spine 19:165–172

140. Hodges P W 1996 Motor control of transversus abdominis for stabilisation of the lumbar spine. PhD Thesis, Department of Physiotherapy, The University of Queensland

141. Hodges P W, Butler J E, McKenzie D, Gandevia S C 1997 Contraction of the human diaphragm during postural adjustments. Journal of Physiology 505:239–548

142. Hodges P W, Cresswell A G, Thorstensson A 1998 Complex preparatory trunk motion around three orthogonal axes precedes asymmetrical upper limb movement. (Submitted)

143. Hodges P W, Cresswell A G, Thorstensson A 1998 Feedforward postural activation of the trunk muscles is altered by arm afferents. (Submitted)

144. Hodges P W, Cresswell A G, Thorstensson A 1998 Preparatory trunk motion precedes upper limb movement. Experimental brain research (in press)

145. Hodges P W, Gandevia S C, Richardson C A 1997 Contractions of specific abdominal muscles in postural tasks are affected by respiratory maneuvers. Journal of Applied Physiology 83:753–760

146. Hodges P W, Richardson C A 1996 Inefficient muscular stabilisation of the lumbar spine associated with low back pain: a motor control evaluation of transversus abdominis. Spine 21:2640–2650

147. Hodges P W, Richardson C A 1997 Contraction of the abdominal muscles associated with movement of the lower limb. Physical Therapy 77:132–144

148. Hodges P W, Richardson, C A 1997 Feedforward contraction of transversus abdominis is not influenced by the direction of arm movement. Experimental Brain Research 114:62–370

149. Hodges P W, Richardson C A 1997 Relationship between limb movement speed and associated contraction of the trunk muscles. Ergonomics 40:1220–1230

150. Hodges P W, Richardson C A 1998 Delayed postural contraction of transversus abdominis in low back pain associated with movement of the lower limbs. Journal of Spinal Disorders 11:46–56

151. Hodges P W, Richardson C A 1998 Changes in the

central nervous system organisation of transversus abdominis contraction associated with limb movement. (Submitted)

152. Hodges P W, Richardson C A 1998 Transversus abdominis and the superficial abdominal muscles are controlled independently in a postural task. (Submitted)

153. Hodges P W, Richardson C A, Jull G A 1996 Evaluation of the relationship between the findings of a laboratory and clinical test of transversus abdominis function. Physiotherapy Research International 1:30–40

154. Hoffer J, Andreassen S 1981 Regulation of soleus muscle stiffness in premamillary cats. Journal of Neurophysiology 45:267–285

155. Hollinshead W H, Jenkins D B 1981 Functional anatomy of the limbs and back. W B Saunders, Philadelphia

156. Holm S, Nachemson A 1983 Variations in the nutrition of the canine intervertebral disc induced by motion. Spine 8:866–874

157. Hongo T, Jankowska E, Lundberg A 1969 The rubrospinal tract II. Facilitation of interneuronal transmission in reflex paths to motoneurones. Experimental Brain Research 7:365–391

158. Horak F B, Esselman P, Anderson M E, Lynch M K 1984 The effects of movement velocity, mass displaced, and task certainty on associated postural adjustments made by normal and hemiplegic individuals. Journal of Neurology, Neurosurgery and Psychiatry 47:1020–1028

159. Hultman G, Nordin M, Saraste H, Ohlsen H 1993 Body composition, endurance, strength, cross-sectional area and density of mm erector spinae in men with and without low back pain. Journal of Spinal Disorders 6:114–123

160. Hurley M V, Newham D J 1993 The influence of arthrogenous muscle inhibition on quadriceps inhibition with quadriceps rehabilitation of patients with early unilateral osteoarthritic knees. British Journal of Rheumatology 32:127–131

161. Isernhagen S J (ed) 1992 Orthopaedic physical therapy clinics of North America: industrial physical therapy. W B Saunders, Philadelphia, vol 1, p 1

162. Janda V 1978 Muscles, central nervous motor regulation and back problems. In: Korr I M (ed) The neurobiologic mechanisms in manipulative therapy. Plenum Press, New York, pp 27–41

163. Janda V 1996 Evaluation of muscular imbalance. In: Liebenson C (ed) Rehabilitation of the spine: a practitioner's manual. Williams & Wilkins, Baltimore, pp 97–112

164. Jayson M, Dixon A 1970 Intra-articular pressure in rheumatoid arthritis of the knee. III. Pressure changes during joint use. Annals of the Rheumatic Diseases 29:401–408

165. Johansson H, Sjolander P, Sojka P 1991 Receptors in the knee joint ligaments and their role in the biomechanics of the joint. CRC Critical Reviews in Biomedical Engineering 18:341–368

166. Johansson H, Sjolander P, Sojka P 1991 A sensory role for the cruciate ligaments. Clinical Orthopaedics and Related Research 268:161–178

167. Johansson H, Sojka P 1991 Pathophysiological mechanisms involved in genesis and spread of muscular tension in occupational muscle pain and in chronic musculoskeletal pain syndromes: a hypothesis. Medical Hypotheses 35:196–203

168. Johnson M A, Polgar J, Weightman D, Appleton D 1973 Data on the distribution of fibre types in thirty-six human muscles: an autopsy study. Journal of the Neurological Sciences 18:111–129

169. Jonsson B 1970 The functions of individual muscles in the lumbar part of the spinae muscle. Electromyography 10:5–21

170. Jorgensen K, Mag C, Nicholaisen T, Kato M 1993 Muscle fibre distribution, capillary density and enzymatic activities in the lumbar paravertebral muscles of young men. Significance for isometric endurance. Spine 18:1439–1450

171. Jorgensen K, Nicolaisen T 1987 Trunk extensor endurance. Determination and relation to low back trouble. Ergonomics 30:259–267

172. Jowett R, Fidler M W, Troup J D G 1975 Histochemical changes in the multifidus in mechanical derangement of the spine. Orthopaedic Clinics of North America 6:145–161

173. Jull G A, Janda V 1986 Muscles and motor control in low back pain: assessment and management. In: Twomey L T, Taylor J (eds) Physical therapy of the low back. Churchill Livingstone, New York, pp 253–278

174. Jull G A, Richardson C A 1994 Rehabilitation of active stabilisation of the lumbar spine. In: Twomey L T, Taylor J (eds) Physical therapy of the lumbar spine, 2nd edn. Churchill Livingstone, New York, pp 251–283

175. Jull G A, Richardson C A, Hamilton C A, Hodges P W, Ng J 1995 Towards the validation of a clinical test for the deep abdominal muscles in back pain patients. In: Proceedings of 9th Biennial Conference of the Manipulative Physiotherapists Association of Australia, Gold Coast. MPAA, St Kilda, Victoria, pp 22–25

176. Jull G, Richardson C, Toppenberg R, Comerford M, Bui B 1993 Towards a measure of active muscle control for lumbar stabilisation. Australian Journal of Physiotherapy 39:187–193

177. Kaigle A M, Holm S H, Hansson T H 1995 Experimental instability in the lumbar spine. Spine 20:421–430

178. Kapanji I A 1974 The physiology of the joints: The trunk and vertebral column. Churchill Livingstone, Edinburgh, vol 3

179. Kawaguchi Y, Matsui H, Tsuji H 1994 Back muscle injury after posterior lumbar spine surgery. Part 2: Histologic and histochemical analyses in humans. Spine 19:2598–2602

180. Kendall F P, McCreary E K 1983 Muscles. Testing and function, 3rd edn. Williams & Wilkins, Baltimore

181. Kennedy B 1980 An Australian program for management of back problems. Physiotherapy 66:108–111

182. Kennedy J C, Alexander I J, Hayes K C 1982 Nerve supply to the knee and its functional significance. The American Journal of Sports Medicine 10:329–335

183. Keshner E A, Allum J H J 1990 Muscle activation patterns coordinating postural stability from head to foot. In: Winters J M, Woo S L-Y (eds) Multiple muscle systems: biomechanics and movement organisation. Springer-Verlag, New York, pp 481–497

184. King J C, Lehmkuhl D L, French J, Dimitrijevic M 1988 Dynamic postural reflexes: comparison in normal subjects and patients with chronic low back pain. Current Concepts in Rehabilitation Medicine 4:7–11

185. Kippers V, Parker A W 1984 Posture related to myoelectric silence of erectores spinae during trunk flexion. Spine 7:740–745

186. Kippers V, Parker A W 1985 Electromyographic studies of erectores spinae: symmetrical postures and sagittal trunk motion. Australian Journal of Physiotherapy 31:91–105

187. Kleinrensink G J, Stoeckart R, Meulstee J et al 1994 Lowered motor conduction velocity of the peroneal nerve after inversion trauma. Medicine and Science in Sports and Exercise 26:877–883

188. Klein-Vogelbach S 1991 Therapeutic exercise in functional kinetics. Springer-Verlag, Berlin

189. Knott M, Voss D E 1968 Proprioceptive neuromuscular facilitation, 2nd edn. Harper & Row, New York

190. Koes B W, van Tulder M W, van der Windt D A 1994 The efficacy of back schools: a review of randomised clinical trials. Journal of Clinical Epidemiology 47:851–862

191. Koes B W, van den Hoogen H M 1994 Efficacy of bed rest and orthoses for low back pain: a review of randomised clinical trials. European Journal Physical Medicine and Rehabilitation 4:86–93

192. Koes B, Assendelft W, Heijdeng G van der, Bouter L, Knipschild P 1991 Spinal manipulation and mobilisation for back and neck pain: a blinded review. British Medical Journal 303:1298–1303

193. Koes B W, Assendelft W J, van der Heijden G J, Bouter L M 1996 Spinal manipulation for low back pain: an updated systematic review of randomised clinical trials. Spine 21:2860–2871

194. Koes B W, Bouter L M, Beckerman H, van der Heijden G J, Knipschild P G 1991 Physiotherapy exercises and back pain: a blinded review. British Medical Journal 302:1572–1576

195. Kornecki S 1992 Mechanism of muscular stabilisation process in joints. Journal of Biomechanics 25:235–245

196. Kottke F J, Halpern D, Easton J K M, Ozel A T, Burrill C A 1978 The training of coordination. Archives of Physical Medicine and Rehabilitation 59:567–572

197. Krag M H, Byrne K B, Gilbertson L G, Haugh L D 1986 Failure of intraabdominal pressurization to reduce erector spinae loads during lifting tasks. In: Allard P, Gagnon M (eds) Proceedings of the North American Congress on Biomechanics, pp 87–88

198. Krebs D E, Staples W H, Cuttita D, Zickel R E 1983 Knee joint angle: its relationship to quadriceps femoris in normal and post arthrotomy limbs. Archives of Physical Medicine and Rehabilitation 64:441–447

199. Kumar S 1980 Physiological responses to weight lifting in different planes. Ergonomics 23:987–993

200. Kuno M 1984 A hypothesis for neural control of the speed of muscle contraction in the mammal. Advances in Biophysics 17:69–95

201. Laasonen E M 1984 Atrophy of sacrospinal muscle groups in patients with chronic diffusely radiating lumbar back pain. Neuroradiology 26:9–13

202. Lacôte M, Clevalier A M, Mirander A, Bleton J P, Stevenin P 1987 Clinical evaluation of muscle function. Churchill Livingstone, Edinburgh

203. Latash M L, Aruin A S, Neyman I, Nichols J J 1995 Anticipatory postural adjustments during self inflicted and predictable perturbations in Parkinson's disease. Journal of Neurology, Neurosurgery and Psychiatry 58:326–334

204. Lavender S A, Mirka G A, Schoenmarklin R W, Sommerich C M, Sudhakar L R, Marras W S 1989 The effects of preview and task symmetry on trunk muscle response to sudden loading. Human Factors 31:101–115

205. Lavender S A, Tsuang Y-H, Hafezi A, Andersson G B J, Chaffin D B, Hughes R E 1992 Coactivation of the trunk muscles during asymmetric loading of the torso. Human Factors 34:239–247

206. Lee W A 1980 Anticipatory control of postural and task muscles during rapid arm flexion. Journal of Motor Behaviour 12:185–196

207. Lee W A, Buchanan T S, Rogers M W 1987 Effects of arm acceleration and behavioural conditions on the organisation of postural adjustments during arm flexion. Experimental Brain Research 66:257–270

208. Lennon S 1982 The Bobath concept: a critical review of the theoretical assumptions that guide physiotherapy practice in stroke rehabilitation. Physical Therapy Review 1:35–45

209. Lewin T, Moffett B, Viidik A 1962 The morphology of the lumbar synovial joints. Acta Morphologica Neerlando Scandinavica 4:299–319

210. Lieb F J, Perry J 1968 An anatomical and mechanical study using amputated limbs. Journal of Bone and Joint Surgery 50A:1535–1548

211. Lieb F J, Perry J 1971 Quadriceps function. Journal of Bone and Joint Surgery 53A:749–758

212. Lund J P, Donga R, Widmer C G, Stohler C S 1991 The pain-adaption model: a discussion of the relationships between chronic musculoskeletal pain and motor activity. Canadian Journal of Physiology and Pharmacology, 69:683–694

213. Lundberg A, Malmgren K, Schomburg E D 1978 Role of joint afferents in motor control exemplified by effects on reflex pathways from 1b afferents. Journal of Physiology 284:327–343

214. Luoto S, Hurri H, Alaranta H 1995 Reaction time in patients with chronic low back pain. European Journal of Physical Medicine and Rehabilitation 5:47–50

215. Lutz G E, Palmitier R A, Chao E Y S 1993 Comparison of tibiofemoral joint forces during open-kinetic-chain and closed kinetic chain exercises. The Journal of Bone and Joint surgery 75A:732–739

216. McCloskey D I 1978 Kinesthetic sensibility. Physiological Review 58:763–820

217. McConnell J 1993 Promoting effective segmental alignment. In: Crosbie J, McConnell J (eds) Key issues in musculoskeletal physiotherapy. Butterworths, London, pp 172–194

218. McGill S M 1991 Electromyographic activity of the abdominal and low back musculature during the generation of isometric and dynamic axial trunk torque: implications for lumbar mechanics. Journal of Orthopaedic Research 9:91–103

219. McGill S M 1991 Kinetic potential of the lumbar trunk musculature about three orthogonal orthopaedic axes in extreme postures. Spine 16:809–815

220. McGill S M 1996 A revised anatomical model of the abdominal musculature for torso flexion efforts. Journal of Biomechanics 29:973–977

221. McGill S M, Juker D, Kropf P 1996 Quantitative intramuscular myoelectric activity of quadratus lumborum during a wide variety of tasks. Clinical Biomechanics 11:170–172

222. McGill S M, Norman R W 1987 Reassessment of the role of intra-abdominal pressure in spinal compression. Ergonomics 30:1565–1588

223. McGill S M, Norman R W 1988 Potential of lumbodorsal fascia forces to generate back extension moments in squat lifts. Journal of Biomedical Engineering 10:312–318

224. McGill S M, Norman R W 1993 Low back biomechanics in industry: the prevention of injury through safer lifting. In: Grabiner M D (ed) Current issues in biomechanics. Human Kinetics, Champaign, Illinois, pp 69–120

225. McGill S M, Norman R W, Sharratt M T 1990 The effect of an abdominal belt on trunk muscles activity and intra-abdominal pressure during squat lifts. Ergonomics 33:147–160

226. McGill S M, Sharratt M T 1990 Relationship between intra-abdominal pressure and trunk EMG. Clinical Biomechanics 5:59–67

227. Macintosh J E, Bogduk N 1986 The morphology of the lumbar erector spinae. Spine 12:658–668

228. Macintosch J E, Bogduk N, Gracovetsky S 1987 The biomechanics of the thoracolumbar fascia. Clinical Biomechanics 2:78–83

229. Macintosh J E, Pearcy M J, Bogduk N 1993 The axial torque of the lumbar back muscles. Australia and New Zealand Journal of Surgery 63:205–212

230. Macintosh J E, Valencia F, Bogduk N, Munro R R 1986 The morphology of the human lumbar multifidus. Clinical Biomechanics 1:196–204

231. Mackenzie M E, Ng G Y 1995 Investigation of progressive high speed non-weight-bearing exercise to triceps surae. New Zealand Journal of Physiotherapy, August p 17–19

232. Mairiaux P, Davis P R, Subbs D A, Baty D 1984 Relation between intra-abdominal pressure and lumbar movements when lifting weights in the erect posture. Ergonomics 27:883–894

233. Marras W, Joynt R L, King A I 1985 The force velocity relation and intra-abdominal pressure during lifting activities. Ergonomics 28:603–613

234. Marras W S, Mirka G A 1990 Muscle activities during asymmetric trunk angular accelerations. Journal of Orthopaedic Research 8:824–832

235. Marras W S, Mirka G A 1996 Intra-abdominal pressure during trunk extension motions. Clinical Biomechanics 11:267–274

236. Marras W S, Rangarajulu S L, Lavender S A 1987 Trunk loading and expectation. Ergonomics 30:551–562

237. Martin J G, DeTroyer A 1982 The behaviour of the abdominal muscles during inspiratory mechanical loading. Respiration Physiology 50:63–73

238. Massion J, Meulders M, Colle J. 1960 Fonction posturale des muscles respiratoires. Archives of International Physiology and Biochemistry 68:314–326

239. Mattila M, Hurme M, Alaranta H et al 1986 The multifidus muscle in patients with lumbar disc herniation. A histochemical and morphometric analysis of intraoperative biopsies. Spine 11:732–738

240. Mayer T G, Vanharanta H, Gatchel R J, Mooney V, Barnes D, Judge L, Smith S 1989 Comparison of CT scan muscle measurements and isokinetic trunk strength in postoperative patients. Spine 14:33–36

241. Mayoux-Benhamou M A, Revel M, Vallee C, Vallee C,

Roudier J P, Bargy F 1994 Longus colli has a postural function of cervical curvature. Surgical and Radiologic Anatomy 16:367–371

242. Miller M I, Medeiros J M 1987 Recruitment of internal oblique and transversus abdominis muscles during the eccentric phase of the curl-up exercise. Physical Therapy 1213–1217

243. Mines A H 1993 Respiratory physiology. Raven, New York

244. Mirka G A, Marras W S 1993 A stochastic model of trunk muscle coactivation during trunk bending. Spine 18:1396–1409

245. Monster A W, Chan H C, O'Connor D 1978 Activity patterns of human skeletal muscles: relation to muscle fibre type composition. Science 200:314–317

246. Monteau R, Hilaire G 1991 Spinal respiratory motoneurons. Progress in Neurobiology 36:83–144

247. Moritani T, DeVries H A 1979 Neural factors versus hypertrophy in the time course of muscle strength gain. American Journal of Physical Medicine 58:115–130

248. Morris J M, Benner F, Lucas D B 1962 An electromyographic study of the intrinsic muscles of the back in man. Journal of Anatomy 96:509–520

249. Morris J M, Lucas D M, Bresler B 1961 Role of the trunk in stability of the spine. Journal of Bone and Joint Surgery 43A:327–351

250. Morrissey M C 1989 Reflex inhibition of thigh muscles in knee injury: causes and treatment. Sports Medicine 7:263–276

251. Nachemson A, Andersson G, Schultz A 1986 Valsalva manoeuvre biomechanics. Effects on lumbar trunk loads of elevated intra-abdominal pressures. Spine 11:456–462

252. Ng G, Richardson C A 1990 The effects of training triceps using progressive speed loading. Physiotherapy Practice 6:77–84

253. Ng J K-F, Kippers V, Richardson C A 1998 Muscle fibre orientation of human abdominal muscles and placement of surface EMG electrodes. Electromyography and Clinical Neurophysiology 38:51–58

254. Nicolaisen T, Jorgensen K 1985 Trunk strength, back muscle endurance and low back trouble. Scandinavian Journal of Rehabilitation Medicine 17:121–127

255. Nielson J, Kagamihara Y 1992 The regulation of disynaptic reciprocal 1a inhibition during co-contraction of antagonistic muscles in man. Journal of Physiology 456:373–393

256. Nouwen A, Van Akkerveeken P F, Versloot J M 1987 Patterns of muscular activity during movement in patients with chronic low back pain. Spine 12:777–782

257. O'Sullivan P B, Twomey L T, Allison G T 1997 Evaluation of specific stabilizing exercise in the treatment of chronic low back pain with radiologic diagnosis of spondylolysis or spondylolisthesis. Spine 22:2959–2967

258. O'Sullivan P, Twomey L, Allison G 1997 Altered pattern of abdominal muscle activation in chronic back pain patients. Australian Journal of Physiotherapy 43:91–98

259. O'Sullivan P B, Twomey L T, Allison G T, Taylor J 1997 Specific stabilising exercise in the treatment of chronic low back pain with a clinical and radiological diagnosis of lumbar segmental 'instability'. In: Proceedings, 10th Biennial Conference Manipulative Physiotherapists

Association of Australia Conference, Melbourne. MPAA, St Kilda, Melbourne, pp. 139–140

260. Oxland T R, Panjabi M M 1992 The onset and progression of spinal instability: a demonstration of neutral zone sensitivity. Journal of Biomechanics 25:1165–1172

261. Pal'tsev Y I, El'ner A N 1967 Preparatory and compensatory period during voluntary movement in patients with involvement of the brain of different localisation. Biofizika 12:142–147

262. Panjabi M M 1992 The stabilising system of the spine. Part 1. Function, dysfunction, adaption, and enhancement. Journal of Spinal Disorders 5:383–389

263. Panjabi M 1992 The stabilising system of the spine. Part II. Neutral zone and stability hypothesis. Journal of Spinal Disorders 5:390–397

264. Panjabi M M 1994 Lumbar spine instability: a biomechanical challenge. Current Orthopaedics 8:100–105

265. Panjabi M, Abumi K, Duranceau J, Oxland T 1989 Spinal stability and intersegmental muscle forces. A biomechanical model. Spine 14:194–200

266. Parkhurst T M, Burnett C N 1994 Injury and proprioception in the lower back. Journal of Orthopaedic and Sports Physical Therapy 19:282–295

267. Parkkola R, Rytokoski U, Kormano M 1993 Magnetic resonance imaging of the discs and trunk muscles in patients with chronic low back pain and healthy control subjects. Spine 18:830–836

268. Parnianpour M, Nordin M, Kahanovitz N, Frankel V 1988 The triaxial coupling of torque generation of trunk muscles during isometric exertions and the effect of fatiguing isoinertial movements on the motor output and movement patterns. Spine 13:982–992

269. Partridge M J, Walters C E 1959 Participation of abdominal muscles in various movements of the trunk in man: an electromyographic study. Physical Therapy Review 39:791–800

270. Pauly J E 1966 An electromyographic analysis of certain movements and exercises: some deep muscles of the back. The Anatomical Record 155:223–234

271. Pope M H, Johnson R J, Brown D W, Tighe C 1979 The role of the musculature in injuries to the medial collateral ligament. Journal of Bone and Joint Surgery 61A:398–402

272. Pope M H, Panjabi M M 1985 Biomechanical definitions of instability. Spine 10:255–256

273. Porterfield J A, DeRosa C 1991 Mechanical low back pain: Perspectives in functional anatomy. W B Saunders, Philadelphia

274. Rantanen J, Hurme M, Falck B et al 1993 The lumbar multifidus muscle five years after surgery for a lumbar intervertebral disc herniation. Spine 18:568–574

275. Raschke U, Chaffin D B 1996 Trunk and hip muscle recruitment in response to external anterior lumbosacral shear and moment loads. Clinical Biomechanics 3:145–152

276. Regen D M, Anversa P, Capasso J M 1993 Segmental calculation of left ventricular wall stress. American Journal of Physiology 264:H1411–H1421

277. Richardson C A 1987 Investigations into the optimal approach to exercise for the knee musculature. PhD Thesis, Department of Physiotherapy, The University of Queensland

278. Richardson C 1987 Atrophy of vastus medialis in patello-femoral pain syndrome. In: Proceedings Tenth International Congress World Confederation for Physical Therapy, Sydney, pp 400–403

279. Richardson C A, Bullock M I 1986 Changes in muscle activity during fast, alternating flexion-extension movements of the knee. Scandinavian Journal of Rehabilitation Medicine 18:51–58

280. Richardson C A, Jull G A 1994 Concepts of rehabilitation for spinal stability. In: Boyling J D, Palastanga N (eds) Grieves modern manual therapy, 2nd edn. Churchill Livingstone, Edinburgh, pp 705–720

281. Richardson C A, Jull G A 1995 Muscle control – pain control. What exercises would you prescribe? Manual Therapy 1:2–10

282. Richardson C A, Jull G A, Richardson B A 1995 A dysfunction of the deep abdominal muscles exists in low back pain patients. In: Proceedings World Confederation of Physical Therapists, Washington, p 932

283. Richardson C, Jull G, Toppenberg R, Comerford M 1992 Techniques for active lumbar stabilisation for spinal protection. Australian Journal of Physiotherapy 38:105–112

284. Richardson C, Sims K 1991 An inner range holding contraction: an objective measure of stabilizing function of an anti-gravity muscle. In: Proceedings of XI Congress of World Confederation of Physical Therapy, London p 829–831

285. Richardson C, Toppenberg R, Jull G 1990 An initial evaluation of eight abdominal exercises for their ability to provide stabilisation for the lumbar spine. Australian Journal of Physiotherapy 36:6–11

286. Rimmer K P, Ford G T, Whitelaw W A 1995 Interaction between postural and respiratory control of human intercostal muscles. Journal of Applied Physiology 79:1556–1561

287. Rizk N N 1980 A new description of the anterior abdominal wall in man and mammals. Journal of Anatomy 131:373–385

288. Robison R 1992 The new back school prescription: Stabilisation training. Part 1. Occupational Medicine 7:17–31

289. Rogers M W, Kukulka C G, Soderberg G L 1987 Postural adjustments preceding rapid arm movements in Parkinsonian subjects. Neuroscience Letters 75:246–251

290. Roy S H, DeLuca C J, Casavant D A 1989 Lumbar muscle fatigue and chronic low back pain. Spine 14:992–1001

291. Roy S H, DeLuca C J, Snyder-Mackler L, Emley M S, Crenshaw R L, Lyons J P 1990 Fatigue, recovery and low back pain in varsity rowers. Medicine and Science in Sports and Exercise 22:463–469

292. Saal J A 1990 Dynamic muscular stabilization in the non-operative treatment of lumbar syndromes. Orthopaedic Review 19:691–700

293. Saal J A, Saal J S 1989 Nonoperative treatment of herniated lumbar intervertebral disc with radiculopathy. An outcome study. Spine 14:431–437

294. Sahrmann S A 1987 Muscle imbalances in the orthopaedic and neurological patient. In: Proceedings of Tenth International Congress of the World Confederation for Physical Therapy, Book, Sydney 2:836–841

295. Sahrmann S 1990 Diagnosis and treatment of muscle imbalances associated with regional pain syndromes. Course notes, Brisbane. Copyright S A Sahrmann, Washington University, School of Medicine, Physical Therapy Department

296. Santavirta S 1979 Integrated Electromyography of the vastus medialis muscle after meniscectomy. American Journal of Sports Medicine 7:40–42

297. Sapsford R, Bullock-Saxton J, Markwell S (eds) 1998 Women's health: a textbook for physiotherapists. W B Saunders, London

298. Sapsford R R, Hodges P W, Richardson C A 1997 Activation of the abdominal muscles is a normal response to contraction of the pelvic floor muscles. International Continence Society Conference, Japan, abstract

299. Sapsford R R, Hodges P W, Richardson C A, Cooper D A, Jull G A, Markwell S J 1997 Activation of pubococcygeus during a variety of isometric abdominal exercises. International Continence Society Conference, Japan, abstract

300. Schmidt R A 1988 Motor control and learning: a behavioural emphasis. Human Kinetics, Champaign, IL

301. Schiable H G, Grubb B D 1993 Afferent and spinal mechanisms of joint pain. Pain 55:5–54

302. Schultz A, Andersson G, Örtengren R, Haderspeck K, Nachemson A 1982 Loads on the lumbar spine. Journal of Bone and Joint Surgery 64A:713–720

303. Sears T A 1964 The slow potentials of thoracic respiratory motoneurones and their relation to breathing. Journal of Physiology 175:404–424

304. Shekelle P, Adams A, Chassin M, Hurwitz E, Brook R 1992 Spinal manipulation for low back pain. Annals of Internal Medicine 17:590–653

305. Shepherd R, Carr J 1998 Neurological rehabilitation: optimizing motor performance. Butterworth Heinemann, Oxford

306. Sihvonen T, Herno A, Paljarvi L, Airaksinen O, Partanen J, Tapaninaho A 1993 Local denervation atrophy of paraspinal muscles in postoperative failed back syndrome. Spine 18:575–581

307. Sihvonen T, Partanen J, Hanninen O, Soimakallio S 1991 Electric behaviour of low back muscles during lumbar pelvic rhythm in low back pain patients and healthy controls. Archives of Physical Medicine and Rehabilitation 72:1080–1087

308. Simmons R W, Richardson C 1992 Peripheral control of the antagonist muscle during unexpectedly loaded arm movements. Brain Research 585:260–266

309. Sinderby C, Ingvarsson P, Sullivan L, Wickstrom I, Lindstrom L 1992 The role of the diaphragm in trunk extension in tetraplegia. Paraplegia 30:389–395

310. Sinderby C, Weinberg J, Sullivan L, Lindstrom L, Grassino A 1996 Electromyographical evidence for exercise-induced diaphragm fatigue in patients with chronic cervical cord injury or prior poliomyelitis infection. Spinal Cord 34:594–601

311. Sirca A, Kostevc V 1985 The fibre type composition of thoracic and lumbar paravertebral muscles in man. Journal of Anatomy 141:131–137

312. Snijders C J, Vleeming A, Stoekart R, Mens J M A, Kleinrensink G J 1995 Biomechanical modeling of sacroiliac joint stability in different postures. Spine: State of the Art Reviews. Hanley & Belfus, Philadelphia

313. Snyder-Mackler L, Ladin Z, Schepsis A A, Young J C 1991 Electrical stimulation of the thigh muscles after reconstruction of the anterior cruciate ligament. Journal of Bone and Joint Surgery 73A:1025–1036

314. Soderberg G L, Barr J O 1983 Muscular function in chronic low back dysfunction. Spine 8:79–85

315. Soderberg G L, Cook T M 1984 Electromyography in biomechanics. Physical Therapy 64:1813–1820

316. Spencer J D, Hayes K C, Alexander I J 1984 Knee joint effusion and quadriceps reflex inhibition in man. Archives of Physical Medicine and Rehabilitation 65:171–177

317. Steffen R, Nolte L P, Pingel T H 1994 Rehabilitation of postoperative segmental lumbar instability. A biomechanical analysis of the rank of the back muscles. Rehabilitation 33:164–170

318. Stener B 1969 Reflex inhibition of the quadriceps elicited from a subperiosteal tumour of the femur. Acta Orthopaedica Scandinavica 40:86–91

319. Stokes M, Cooper R 1993 Physiological factors influencing performance of skeletal muscle. In: Crosbie J, McConnell J (eds) Key issues in musculoskeletal physiotherapy. Butterworth Heinemann, Oxford

320. Stokes M J, Hides J A, Jull G A, Cooper D H 1992 Mechanism of human paraspinal wasting with acute low back pain. Journal of Physiology 452:280P

321. Stokes M, Hides J, Nassiri K 1997 Musculoskeletal ultrasound imaging: diagnostic and treatment aid in rehabilitation. Physical Therapy Reviews 2:73–92

322. Stokes M, Young A 1984 The contribution of reflex inhibition to arthrogenous muscle weakness. Clinical Science 67:7–14

323. Stokes M, Young A 1984 Investigations of quadriceps inhibition: implications for clinical practice. Physiotherapy 70:425–428

324. Stratford P 1981 EMG of the quadriceps femoris muscles in subjects with normal knees and acutely effused knees. Physical Therapy 62:279–283

325. Strohl K P, Mead J, Banzett R B, Loring S H, Kosch P C 1981 Regional differences in abdominal muscle activity during various manoeuvres in humans. Journal of Applied Physiology 51:1471–1476

326. Sullivan P E, Markus P D 1987 Clinical procedures in therapeutic exercise. Reston Publishing, Reston

327. Taimela S, Österman K, Alaranta H, Soukka A, Kujala U M 1993 Long psychomotor reaction time in patients with chronic low-back pain. Archives of Physical Medicine and Rehabilitation 74:1161–1164

328. Tertti M O, Salminen J J, Paajanen H E K, Terho P H, Kormano M J 1991 Low back pain and disc degeneration in children: a case control MR imaging study. Radiology 180:503–507

329. Tesh K M, ShawDunn J, Evans J H 1987 The abdominal muscles and vertebral stability. Spine 12:501–508

330. Thelen D G, Schultz A B, Ashton-Miller J A 1995 Co-contraction of lumbar muscles during the development of time-varying triaxial moments. Journal of Orthopaedic Research 13:390–398

331. Thompson K D 1997 Estimation of loads and stresses in abdominal muscles during slow lifts. Proceedings of the Institution of Mechanical Engineers 211:271–274

332. Thomson K D 1988 On the bending moment capability of the pressurized abdominal cavity during human lifting activity. Ergonomics 31:817–828

333. Thorstensson A, Carlson H 1987 Fibre types in human lumbar back muscles. Acta Physiologica Scandinavica 131:195–200

334. Thorstensson A, Oddsson L, Carlson H 1985 Motor control of voluntary trunk movements in standing. Acta Physiologica Scandinavica 125:309–321

335. Travell J G, Simons D G 1983 Myofascial pain and dysfunction. The trigger point manual. Williams & Wilkins, Baltimore

336. Troup J D G 1965 Relation of lumbar spine disorders to heavy manual work and lifting. Lancet i:857–861

337. Troup J D G, Leskinen T P J, Stalhammer H R, Kuorinka I A A 1983 A comparison of intraabdominal pressure increases, hip torque, and lumbar vertebral compression in different lifting techniques. Human Factors 25:517–525

338. Uhlig Y, Weber B R, Grob D, Muntener M 1995 Fiber composition and fiber transformations in neck muscles of patients with dysfunction of the cervical spine. Journal of Orthopaedic Research 13:240–249

339. Valencia F P, Munro R R 1985 An electromyographic study of the lumbar multifidus in man. Electromyography and Clinical Neurophysiology 25:205–221

340. Van Ingen Schenau G J, Boots P J M, De Groot G, Snackers R J, van Woensel W W L M 1992 The constrained control of force and position in multijoint movements. Neuroscience 46:197–207

341. Van Tulder M W, Koes B W, Bouter L M 1997 Conservative treatment of acute and chronic low back pain. A systematic review of randomised controlled trials of the most common interventions. Spine 22:2128–2156

342. Venna S, Hurri H, Alaranta H 1994 Correlation between neurological leg deficits and reaction time of upper limbs among low-back pain patients. Scandinavian Journal of Rehabilitation Medicine 26:87–90

343. Verbout A J, Wintzen A R, Linthorst P 1989 The distribution of slow and fast twitch fibres in the intrinsic back muscles. Clinical Anatomy 2:120–121

344. Vitti M, Fujiwara M, Basmajian J, Iida M 1973 The integrated roles of longus colli and sternocleidomastoid muscles: an electromyographic study. The Anatomical Record 177:471–484

345. Vleeming A, Pool-Goudzwaard A L, Stoeckart R, vanWingerden J-P, Snijders C J 1995 The posterior layer of the thoracolumbar fascia: its function in load transfer from spine to legs. Spine 20:753–758

346. Vleeming A, Stoeckart R, Snijders C J 1989 The sacrotuberous ligament: a conceptual approach to its dynamic role in stabilising the sacroiliac joint. Clinical Biomechanics 4:201–203

347. Wakai Y, Welsh M M, Leevers A M, Road J D 1992 Expiratory muscle activity in the awake and sleeping human during lung inflation and hypercapnia. Journal of Applied Physiology 72:881–887

348. Weber B, Uhlig Y, Grob D, Dvorak J, Muntener M 1993 Duration of pain and muscular adaptions in patients with dysfunction of the cervical spine. Journal of Orthopaedic Research 11:805–810

349. Wedin S, Leanderson R, Knutsson E 1987 The effect of voluntary diaphragmatic activation on back lifting. Scandinavian Journal of Rehabilitation Medicine 20:129–132

350. Weiler P J, King G J, Gertzbein S D 1990 Analysis of sagittal plane instability of the lumbar spine in vivo. Spine 15:1300–1306

351. White A A, Panjabi M M 1990 Clinical biomechanics of the spine, 2nd edn. J B Lippincott, Philadelphia

352. White M J, Davies C T M 1984 The effects of immobilisation, after lower leg fracture, on the contractile properties of human triceps surae. Clinical Science 66:277–282

353. White S G, Sahrmann S A 1994 Movement system balance approach to management of musculoskeletal pain. In: Grant R (ed.) Clinics in physical therapy: physical therapy of the cervical and thoracic spine, 2nd edn. Churchill Livingstone, Edinburgh

354. Wilke H J, Wolf S, Claes L E, Arand M, Wiesend A 1995 Stability increase of the lumbar spine with different muscles groups. A biomechanical in vitro study. Spine 20:192–198

355. Williams P L, Warwick R, Dyson M, Bannister L H (eds) 1989 Gray's anatomy, 37th edn. Churchill Livingstone, Edinburgh, pp 592–604

356. Winters J M, Peles J D 1990 Neck muscle activity and 3D head kinematics during quasistatic and dynamic tracking movements. In: Winters J M, Woo S L-Y (eds) Multiple muscle systems: biomechanics and movement organization. Springer-Verlag, New York, pp 461–480

357. Wise H H, Fiebert I M, Kates J L 1984 EMG biofeedback as treatment for patellofemoral pain syndrome. The Journal of Orthopaedic and Sports Physical Therapy 6:95–103

358. Wohlfahrt D A, Jull G A, Richardson C A 1993 An initial investigation of the relationship between the dynamic and static function of the abdominal muscles. Australian Journal of Physiotherapy 39:9–14

359. Wolf E, Magora A, Gonen B 1971 Disuse atrophy of the quadriceps muscle. Electromyography 11:479–490

360. Wolf S L, Basmajian J V, Russe T C, Kutner M 1979 Normative data on low back mobility and activity levels. American Journal of Physical Medicine 58:217–229

361. Woo S L, Winters J M (eds) 1990 Multiple muscle systems. Springer-Verlag, New York

362. Woolf C J, Wall P D 1986 Relative effectiveness of C primary afferent fibres of different origins in evoking a prolonged facilitation of the flexor reflex in the rat. The Journal of Neuroscience 6:1433–1442

363. Zattara M, Bouisset, S 1988 Posturo-kinetic organisation during the early phase of voluntary upper limb movement. I. Normal subjects. Journal of Neurology, Neurosurgery and Psychiatry 51:956–965

364. Zetterberg C, Aniansson, Grimby G 1983 Morphology of the paravertebral muscles in adolescent idiopathic scoliosis. Spine 8:457–462

365. Zhu X Z, Parnianpour M, Nordin M, Kahanovitz N 1989 Histochemistry and morphology of erector spinae muscles in lumbar disc herniation. Spine 14:391–397

# Index